Welcome to ...

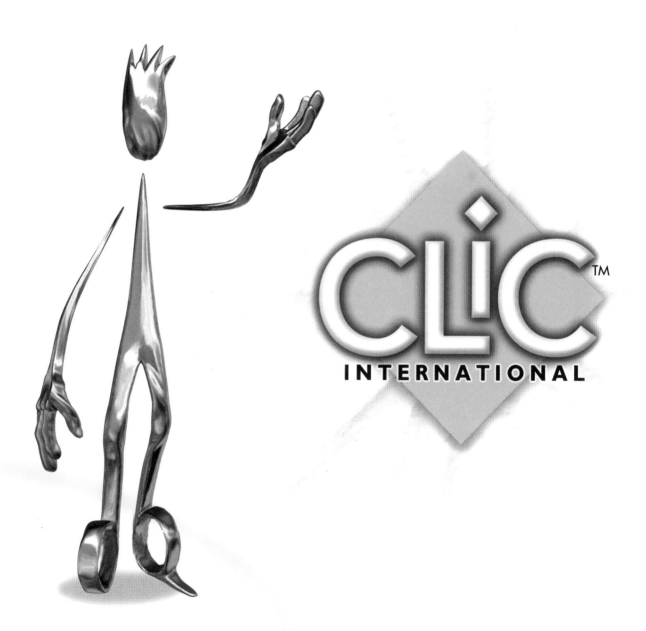

CLiC™
INTERNATIONAL

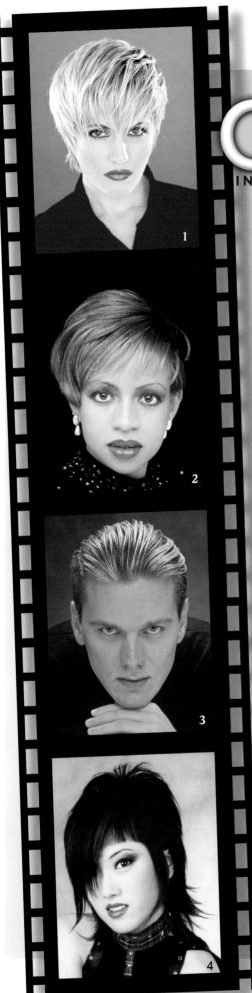

CLiC
INTERNATIONAL

CERTIFIED
LEARNING IN
COSMETOLOGY®

Architecture

haircutting

Architectural
haircutting

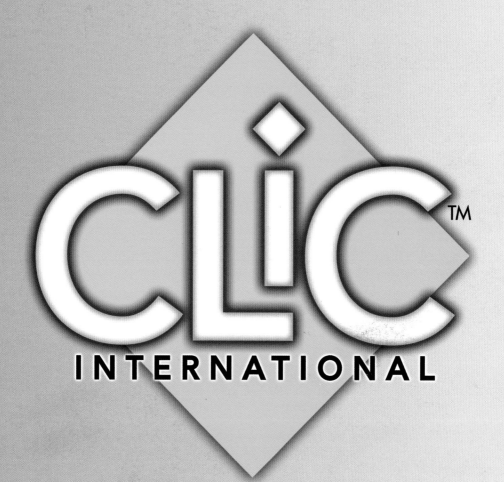

CLiC™
INTERNATIONAL

A Passion for Perfection©

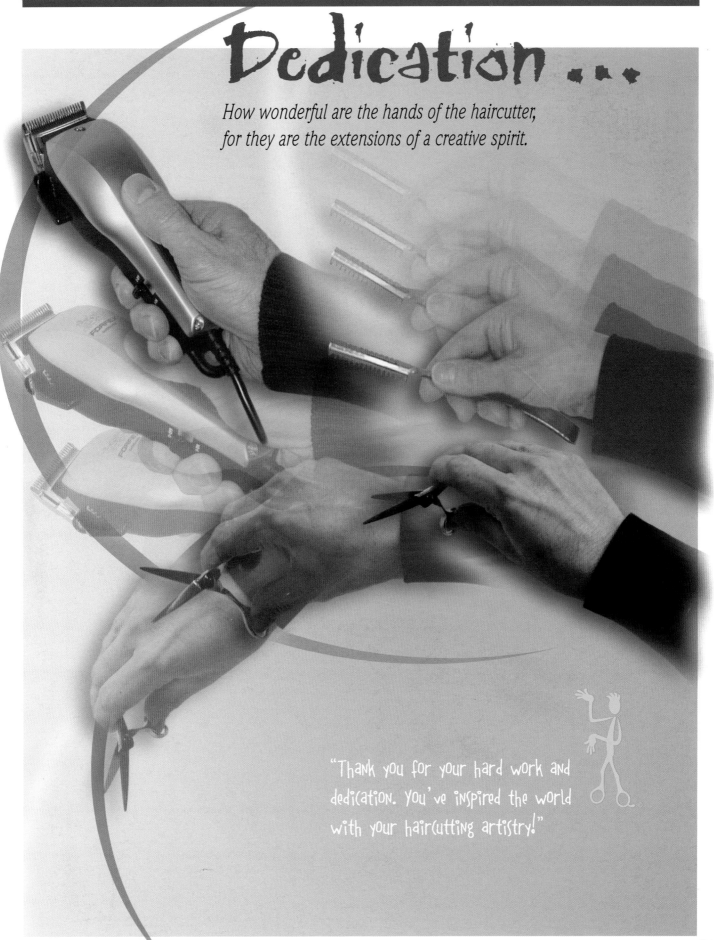

Dedication ...

*How wonderful are the hands of the haircutter,
for they are the extensions of a creative spirit.*

"Thank you for your hard work and
dedication. You've inspired the world
with your haircutting artistry!"

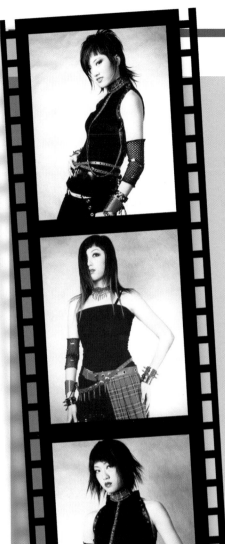

HAIR
Artist page(picture number)

Adam S. Swayne 237(1)
Alberto Oyola 223(3)
Allante Hair Design
191(A1), 192
Antenna Salon & Beyond
1(3), 7(1)
Belinda Baker
26(3), 67(4,5,8), 101(1), 150(3), 214(3), 222(4), 226(3)
All photographs ©2003 Belinda Baker, all rights reserved.

Ben DeCordova
15(1), 17(2), 18(1), 23(2), 60, 106(2), 116(6), 122(2), 142(3,4), 155(A2), 158, 216(4), 219(3)
Beth Boyer 236(1)
BladezSalon.com 144(4)
Blaine Fasnacht 234(3)
Bob Steele Hairdressers
1(1), 67(2,7), 72(1), 103(2,3), 139, 144(3), 146(2), 148(1), 149(3), 150(2), 151(6), 149(3), 212(3), 213(4), 214(4), 215(2), 217(1), 221(4), 227(1), 232(3)
Brenda Petty
23(3), 26(4), 116(9), 155(A1), 156, 191(C2), 202
Brent Borreson for Salon Visage
67(6), 123(5)
Candice Hodges
16(1), 26(6), 106(1), 116(5), 219(1), 227(3)
CC Garrow Salon 236(2)
Chazio's Salon 224(3)
Chris Baran 155(C4), 180
Chris Tse for Sets
100(2), 151(2,3)
Cloud 9 Hair Salon
77(3), 143(5), 151(5)
D. J. Moran for Grund International 151(1)
Darlene's Hair Hut 150(5)
Davina Guido 191(A2), 194
Duncan Lai
1(4), 4, 5, 6, 14, 16(2), 17(1), 18(2), 20(1), 21(3), 22(1), 23(1), 24(1), 27(1,4), 140(3), 146(1), 155(A5), 164, 222(3)
Edie's Styling Center 116(2), 224(1)
Elon Salon
27(2), 140(2), 155(B3), 170, 214(2), 218(3), 224(2,4)

Expressions Hair Salon 213(3), 218(1)
Fay Puopolo 235(1)
Franco Frittelli 145(3)
Gadabout Salon & Spa
103(1), 147(2), 148(2), 150(1)
Gary Charles & Associates 59(1)
Hair Benders International
116(4), 140(6), 142(1), 143(3), 145(2), 149(1), 216(1), 220(4), 222(2), 223(1)
Hair Cuttery / Bubbles, Inc.
67(3), 111, 147(1), 150 (4,6), 237(2)
Hair Reflections 223(2)
Heather Marie for Fringe Variable
123(4)
Identity Salon & Day Spa
141(4), 155(A3), 160
Imma Marino 155(B4), 172
Indola Worldwide Design Team
212(1)
IZEAR / Uptown Hair Design
59(4), 155(C6), 184
Jean-Philippe Pagès for Oro Vision Magazine
155(C8), 188, 189, 228(1,2,3,4)
Jeffrey LaMorte Salon 122(3), 123(3)
Jenniffer & Company 151(7)
Joanne Fanelli 220(3), 221(3)
John C. Simpsin 236 (3)
Kat Spence 155(B2), 168, 223(4)
KC Design Group 191(B1),196
Ladies & Gentlemen Salon & Spa
7(2), 10, 82, 142(5), 145(1), 155(C3), 178, 212(4)
Linda Auricchio 235(2)
London Hair Salon
22(3), 59(3), 72(3), 140(5), 227(4)
Lori Lopez for Wild Orchids Salon
100(1)
Mandy Wadsworth 221(2)
Manuel Rodriguez 24(2)
Maria Adame 235(3)
Maria Norman 144(2)
Michael Christopher Salon
122(1), 226(4)
Michael Miller 144(1)
Michael Rocco
15(4), 26(1), 104, 155(C5), 182, 232(1)
Morris Gargiule 225(4)
Olive Benson
21(5), 26(5), 27(3), 59(2), 112, 140(1), 155(C2), 176, 213(2)
Olivia Hughes 215(1)
Ozzie Rizzo for Renbow

"A special thanks to all the professionals who provided their photo images to support the education of future cosmetologists. These images show the rewards of mastering the artistry of haircutting."

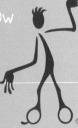

International 134/135
Pamela Boolman 141(2)
Patrick Short 221(1)
Professional Image Salon 151(4)
R Vincent Salon 116(1)
Randy Rick
1(2), 20(2), 22(2,4), 26(2), 27(5), 77(1), 98, 101(2),
141(3), 191 (B2), 198, 218(4), 219(4), 225(1,2),
226(1), 233(3)
Robert Andrew The Salon and Spa 220(2)
Robin Cohen 220(1)
Rose Marie DiCriscio 232(2)
Salon Hazleton 77(2)
Salon Visage 67(1), 116(7)
Sara Aiello 215(4)
Sheer Pleasure by Jeffrey Marshall 217(4)
Sheer Professionals Salon
123(2), 143(2,6), 155(B1), 166, 216(2)
Sherry Gordon Salon 222(1)
Shortino & Friends Salon & Spa 145(5)
Susan Snow 25(2)
Tawny & Company 141(1), 142(2)
Toni & Guy Advanced Hairdressing Academy
www.toniguy.com 217(3)
The Brown Aveda Institute 123(1), 143(1), 151(8)
The Spa at Margo Blue
15(3), 25(1), 155(A4), 162, 225(3)
Timothy Findon 226(2)
Vanis Salon & Spa 143(4), 145(4), 149(2), 217(2)
Victoria Station Salon 219(2)
Vince D'Attilio
25(3), 72(2), 110, 116(3), 148(3), 191(C1), 200,
213(1), 216(3), 233(1), 234(1,2), 237(3)
Xenon 21(2), 215(3)
Yellow Strawberry Global Salon
15(2), 212(2), 214(1), 227(2)

PHOTOGRAPHY
Artist page(picture number)

Andres Aquino 72(4), 113, 155(C1), 174, 233(2)
Archie Carpenter 155(C6), 184
Bambi Cantrel 100(1)
Calvin Childs 16(1), 26(6), 106(1), 116(5), 219(1), 227(3)
Chip Faust www.universalsalons.com 151(4)
Curtis Spratlin
21(5), 26(5), 27(3), 59(2), 112, 140(1), 155(C2),
176, 213(2)
Dan Carter 21(2), 215(3)
Don Nyne 100(2), 151(2,3)
Edward Tytel
23(3), 26(4), 116(9), 155(A1), 156, 191(C2), 202
Ernest Washington 67 (4,5)
Image:www.freeimages.co.uk 140(4)
Insights Technical Cutting Guide
Intra America Beauty Network
www.inspirequarterly.com 217(3)

Jack Cutler
15(4), 21(1), 24(2), 25(2), 26(1), 116(8),
117(1,2,3),141(2), 144(1,2), 145(3),
155(B2,B4, C5,C7), 168, 172, 182, 191(A1), 192,
212(1), 215(1,4), 218(2), 220(1), 221(1,2), 223(4),
225(4), 232(1,2), 234(3), 235(1,2), 236(1)
Jaime Koslow 67(3), 111, 147(1), 150(4,6), 237(2)
John Dalton 21(4), 25(3), 72(2), 191(C1), 200, 233(1)
Jonathan Martin
26(3), 67(8), 101(1), 150(3), 214(3), 222(4),
226(3)
Jonathan Roth 226(2)
Matthew Yates 236 (3)
Photo courtesy of NASA 133(1)
Robert Sargent
15(1), 17(2), 18(1), 23(2), 60, 106(2), 116(6), 122(2),
142(3,4), 155(A2), 158, 216(4), 219(3)
Tom Carson
1(1,2), 7(1,2), 10, 15(2,3), 22(2,3), 25(1), 26(2),
27(2), 59(1,3), 67(1,2,6,7), 72(1,3), 77, 82, 98,
103(2,3), 110, 116(1,2,3,4,7), 122(1,3),
123(1,2,3,5), 140(2,5,6), 141(1,3,4), 142(1,2,5),
143, 144(3,4), 145(1,2,4,5), 146(2), 148(1), 149,
150(2,5), 151(5,5,7,8) 155(A3,A4,B1,B3,C3), 160,
162, 166, 170, 178, 191(A2), 194, 212(2,3,4),
213(1,3,4), 214(1,2,4), 215(2), 216(1,2,3),
217(1,2,4), 218(1,3), 219(2), 220(2,4), 221(4),
222(1,2), 223(1,2), 224, 225(2,3), 226(4),
227(1,2,4), 232(3), 234(2), 236(2), 237(3)
All photographs ©2003 Tom Carson, all rights reserved.
Taggart/Winterhalter for Purely Visual Productions
139, 155(C4), 180
Matthew Yates 236(3)
Cosimo Zaccaria 59(4)

SPECIAL ACKNOWLEDGEMENTS

S.H.E.A.R.S. and C.L.A.S.S.
information on pages 40, 41
Bonnie Megowan www.bonika.com

Director of Education
Margie Wagner

Curriculum Development
Manager
Theresa Ksyniak

Design and Illustration
**CLiC INTERNATIONAL
Art Team**

Condict and Company

Watercolor
LauraGelsomini
204

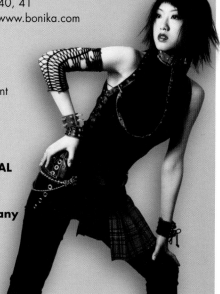

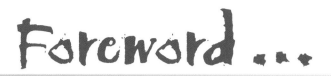
Foreword ...

Sir Isaac Newton once said, "If I have been able to see further, it was only because I stood on the shoulders of giants." This profound statement represents one of the guiding principles of the Certified Learning in Cosmetology® (CLiC) system. There is much to be learned and discovered by "standing on the shoulders of giants." It is only by studying the discoveries and accomplishments of the leaders who came before us that we can prepare for the future.

The CLiC system provides a broad cosmetology education with a focus on three key areas:

1- A basic cosmetology foundation
2- An introduction to artistic concepts and visual
   inspiration to nurture creativity
3- Effective interpersonal, sales and retailing techniques

Although the cosmetology industry is continually evolving, its basic foundation remains unchanged. The foundation of cosmetology is an understanding of human biology combined with scientific and mathematic concepts used to create desired results. Building on the basic foundation of cosmetology, artistic concepts and visual inspiration are then used to develop and nurture creativity. Throughout the foundational and artistic learning process, successful interpersonal, selling and retailing skills are introduced and practiced. These skills are paramount to the financial success of the professional cosmetologist.

You will find CLiC to be a visually exciting and inspirational education system focused on preparing students to be salon ready upon completion of their studies. Developed by an industry giant himself, master hair designer and international award winner Randy Rick is the creative force behind this revolutionary CLiC system. Always a step ahead, Mr. Rick developed the CLiC system of learning to elevate the artistic and practical skills of today's students. Through the CLiC program, he shares his vast international knowledge and experience with you, the cosmetology professional of the future!

CLiC to a dynamic future in haircutting!

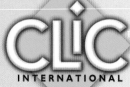

The CLiC Education Team ...

The CLiC Education Team represents more than 100 years of combined cosmetology industry education, experience and wisdom. The team includes international award winners, top educators, stylists, salon and beauty school owners, operations managers and owners and operators of highly successful cosmetology businesses.

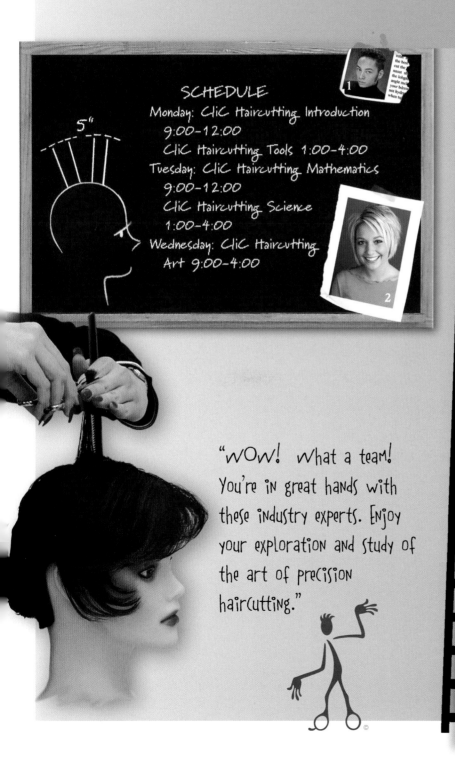

SCHEDULE
Monday: CliC Haircutting Introduction
9:00-12:00
CliC Haircutting Tools 1:00-4:00
Tuesday: CliC Haircutting Mathematics
9:00-12:00
CliC Haircutting Science
1:00-4:00
Wednesday: CliC Haircutting
Art 9:00-4:00

5"

"WOW! What a team! You're in great hands with these industry experts. Enjoy your exploration and study of the art of precision haircutting."

CLiC INTERNATIONAL

CLiC International combines both domestic and internationally accepted principles for each of the key cosmetology arts with salon industry skills. These principles are brought to life from knowledgeable subject matter experts from throughout the world, ranging from industry icons to experienced instructors and artists.

The combination of these key principles presented in a visual story of cosmetology through the talents of our gifted writers, graphic designers and creation team, result in the modern CLiC Visual Learning Education System. This education system is both a stimulating and technically concise unit of learning that enhances the student learning experience, builds a strong foundation for the student to be successful and raises their competency and professionalism to a whole new level.

You are about to begin an exciting journey into the world of cosmetology. The Certified Learning in Cosmetology® (CLiC) system will act as your road map, leading you to reap the rewards of becoming a successful professional cosmetologist.

The CLiC system is designed to enhance the fundamental cosmetology education by incorporating artistic inspiration and successful sales and retail skills. The learning modules cannot possibly cover all fashionable vogues, but will always encourage freedom of expression and innovation to adapt to current trends.

This revolutionary system focuses on meeting your educational needs with a solid, competency-based cosmetology curriculum. Each CLiC module is designed to develop manual dexterity, professional perception, tactile sensitivity and the artistic vision used in the field.

The CLiC educational system is presented in individual learning modules, each a complete program. The module system enables you to focus on individual disciplines within the field by offering courses for certified specialization in each field. This ensures the opportunity to learn and develop the skills needed for a rewarding and profitable career in the cosmetology field of your choice.

For additional information, contact:

CLiC INTERNATIONAL®
396 Pottsville/Saint Clair Highway
Pottsville, PA 17901 USA
1.800.207.5400 USA & Canada
001.570.429.4216 International
1.570.429.4252 Fax
www.clicusa.com

CLiC INTERNATIONAL

CERTIFIED LEARNING IN COSMETOLOGY®

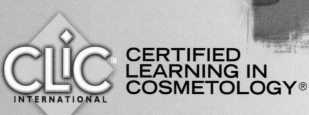

"Explore the work of master artists. It will inspire you and give you a creative edge in your artistic haircutting work."

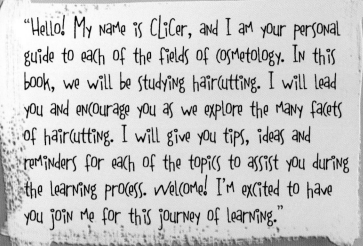

"Hello! My name is CLiCer, and I am your personal guide to each of the fields of cosmetology. In this book, we will be studying haircutting. I will lead you and encourage you as we explore the many facets of haircutting. I will give you tips, ideas and reminders for each of the topics to assist you during the learning process. Welcome! I'm excited to have you join me for this journey of learning."

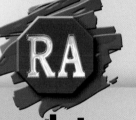

Regulatory Alert

Whenever you see the shadow of the **Regulatory Alert** icon, it will remind you and your instructor to check governmental regulations about the subject on the page. The rules and regulations for cosmetology vary according to geographic location. Place a sticker from the back of the book over the shadow if there are governmental regulations that must be followed in your area.

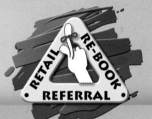

The 3R's

At the conclusion of your services there are three important steps you should consistently follow. **Retail** professional products to your customers for home maintenance. This provides a strong supplement to your income. **Re-book** future appointments to encourage regular visits. Ask for **referrals** to strengthen your customer base. By following the 3R's you will improve your income and profitability as a professional cosmetologist.

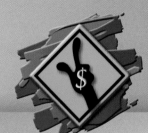

CLiCer's Sales Pointers

As you will learn throughout this book, selling and financial skills will be just as important to your success in the salon as your actual haircutting knowledge and skills. Whenever you see this icon with CLiCer's hand, pay special attention to the **sales pointers** you are given. Combining sales skills with haircutting skills will create a dynamic force for your salon success.

The art of precision haircutting is the foundation to all other hair services performed in the field of cosmetology. It is a highly specialized combination of setting goals, developing technical skills and using creativity and artistic expression.

Your approach to haircutting will be very similar to the architectural approach to designing a building. The two-dimensional blue print of an artistic hair design has limited visual benefits. However, the finished hairdesign becomes an organized architectural structure in three-dimensional form.

The laws of nature must be followed as you engineer the methodology for creating a great haircut, unique to the needs and interests of each individual client. Shapes, proportions and visual relationships should all be considered as you create each haircut.

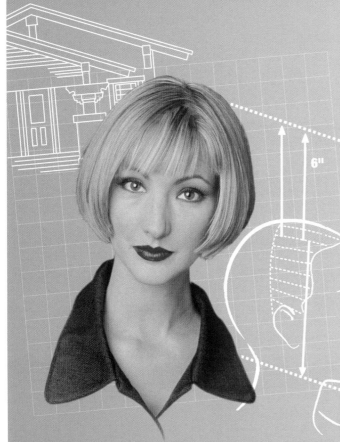

6"

Haircuts have many purposes and benefits, including:

- **to re-shape the fabric of hair**
- **to work easily with a client's lifestyle and activities**
- **to help create a social identity or status**
- **to make a fashion statement**
- **to create a physical expression of oneself**

As a professional haircutting architect, you will create cuts that work well for each client, respond the ways in which they were intended, look great on the client and make an artistically pleasing presentation.

"Remember ... a haircut is only good when it's GREAT!"

Table of Contents ...

"For information about
additional modules, check
out the last page of
this
book."

Inspirational Snippets

"Our greatest glory is not in never falling, but in rising every time we fall."
— Confucius

"From small beginnings come great things."
— Dutch Proverb

"No one can make you feel inferior without your consent."
Eleanor Roosevelt

" Genius is one percent inspiration and ninety-nine percent perspiration. If we all did the things we are capable of doing, we would literally astound ourselves."
— Thomas Edison

'you are an image of your own work'
— Randy Rick

"Do the best work that you can. You never have to apologize for quality."
-Arnold Zegarelli

"Take time to read these 'snippets.' They will inspire you!"

"NEVER UNDERESTIMATE THE POWER OF A GREAT HAIRCUT. IT PROVIDES PEOPLE WITH THE ADDED CONFIDENCE OF KNOWING THEY LOOK GREAT."
— GENO STAMPORA

angle
baseline
boundaries
creativity

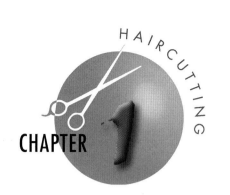

HAIRCUTTING

CHAPTER 1

degree
constructed
stacking

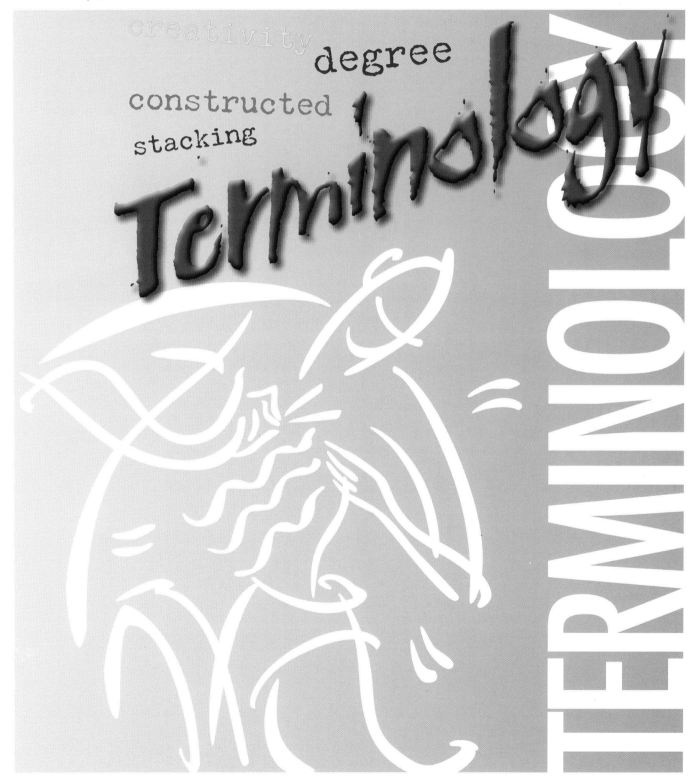

Terminology

TERMINOLOGY

"Mastering the terminology of haircutting is like learning a whole new language.

It will give you the ability to communicate with future clients and fellow professionals. It will also give you a successful edge in your chosen career!"

Abstract

A nonrepresentational design that includes irregular shapes, colors or textures that maintain harmony within the overall form.

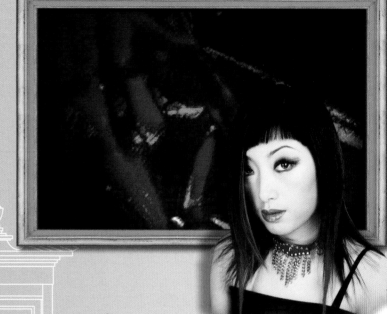

15°

45°

Angle

A measurement of the space between two intersecting lines or planes; measured in degrees.

90°

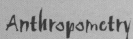

Anthropometry

The study and measurement of the human body and its proportions for examination and comparison purposes.

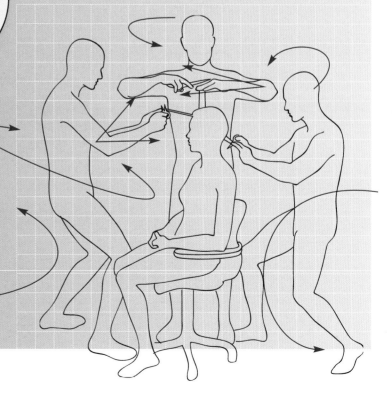

Terminology

Art

Skills and techniques used for creative work and learned by observation, study and hands-on experience.

Balance/Counterbalance

Balance – the harmonious arrangement of the elements of a hair design with nothing emphasized or out of proportion.

Counterbalance – the use of different weights and lengths in opposite areas that offset each other to create a balanced overall appearance.

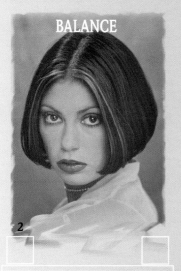

BALANCE

COUNTERBALANCE

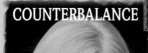

2

3

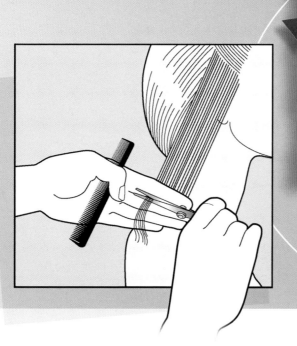

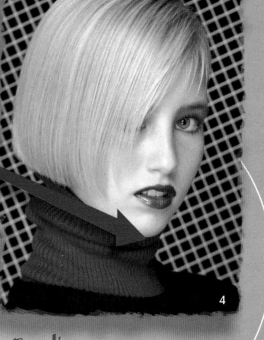

4

Baseline

The perimeter or outer boundary of a haircut; also called a design line or fringe line.

Terminology ...

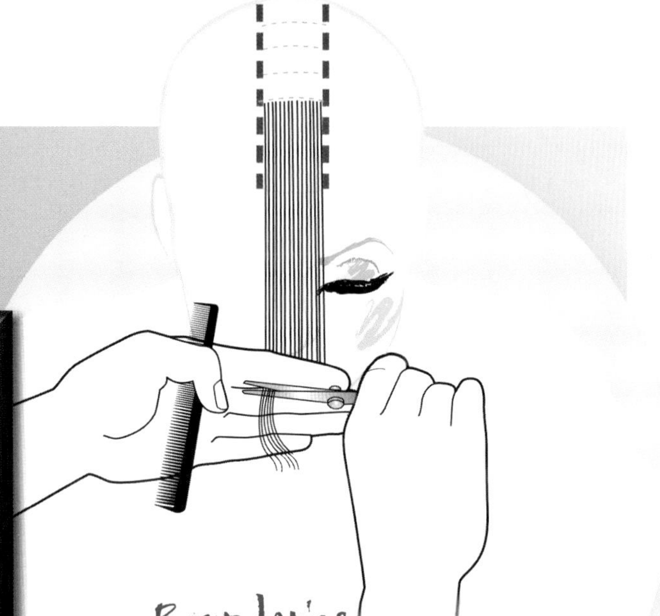

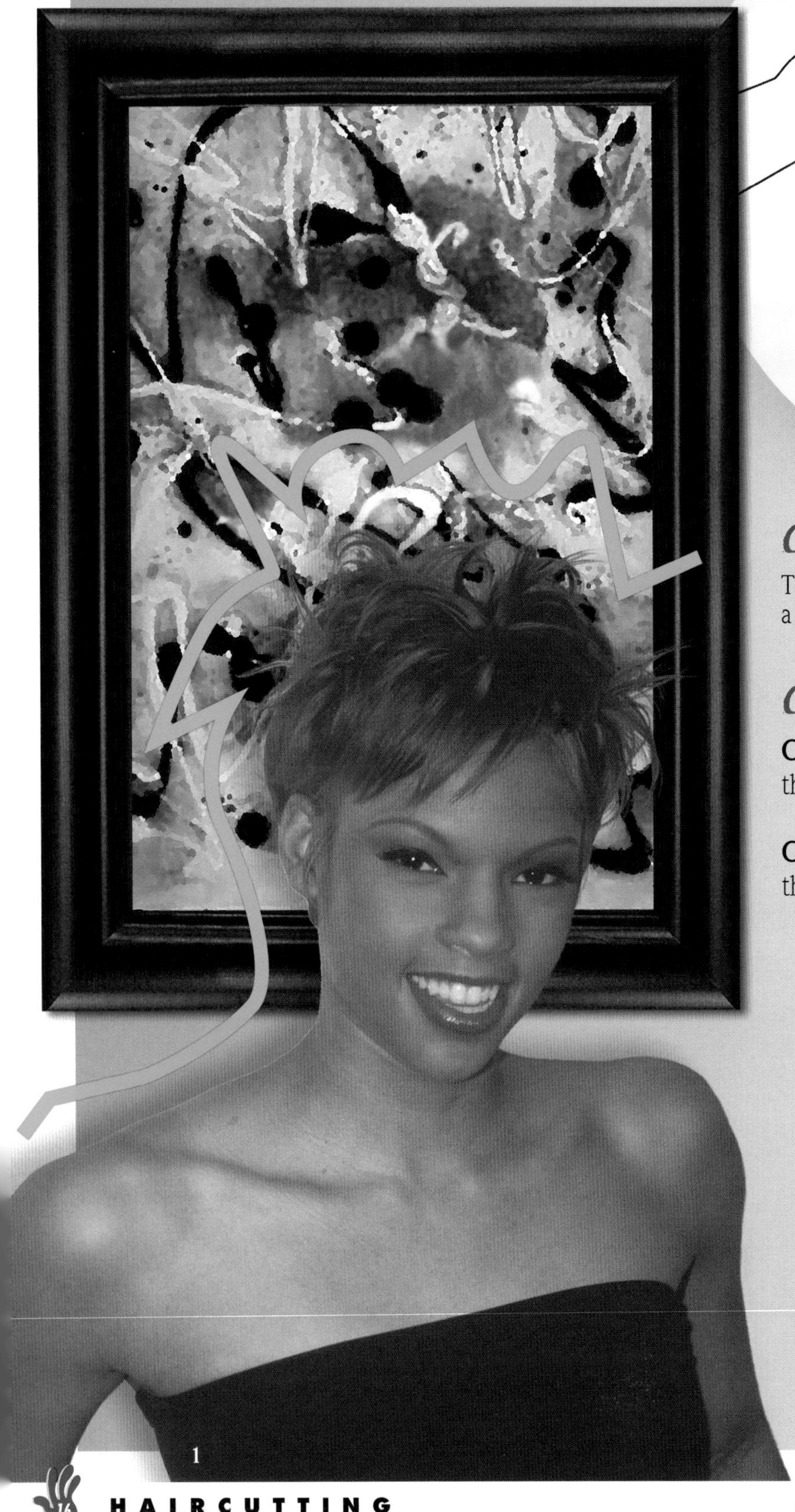

Boundaries

The partings that separate the planes of the head; lines that isolate an area being cut from the rest of the hair.

Commotion

The appearance of motion and excitement in a haircut that is styled in a disorderly fashion.

Concave/Convex

Concave – curving inward; shaped like the inside of a bowl.

Convex – curving outward; shaped like the outside of a sphere.

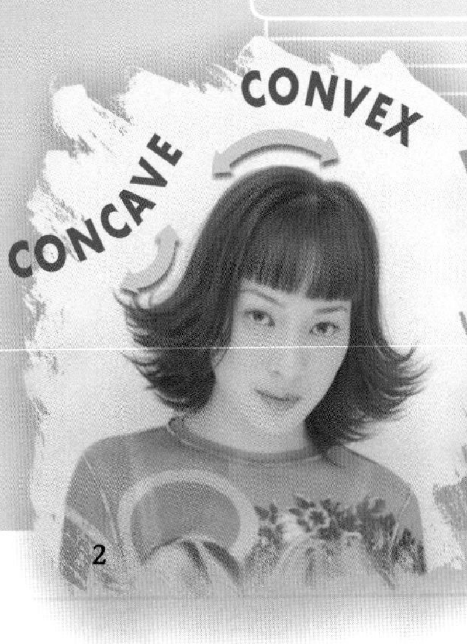

CONCAVE   CONVEX

1

2

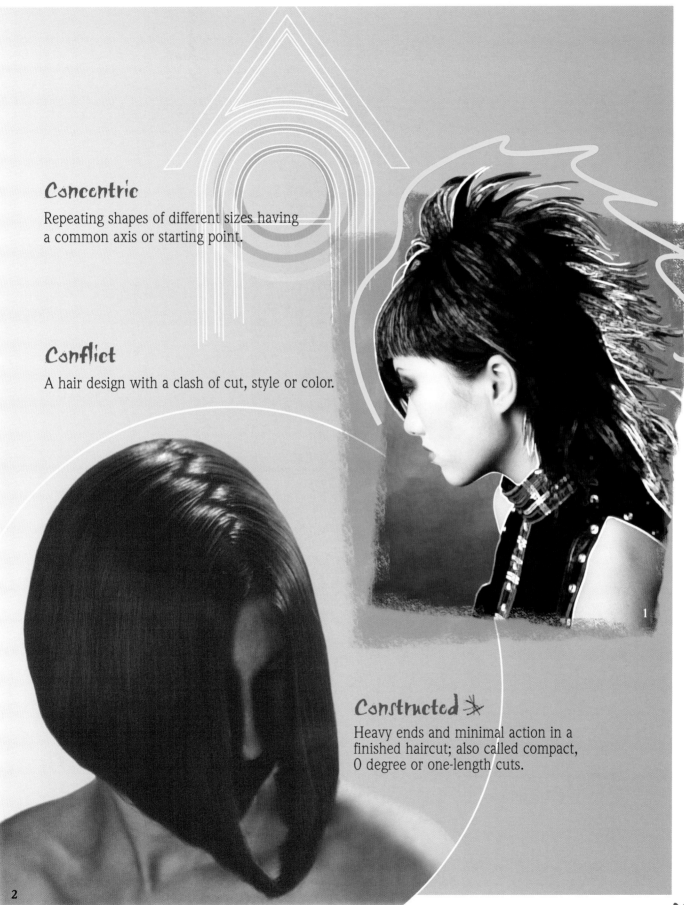

Concentric

Repeating shapes of different sizes having a common axis or starting point.

Conflict

A hair design with a clash of cut, style or color.

Constructed ✳

Heavy ends and minimal action in a finished haircut; also called compact, 0 degree or one-length cuts.

2

1

Terminology ...

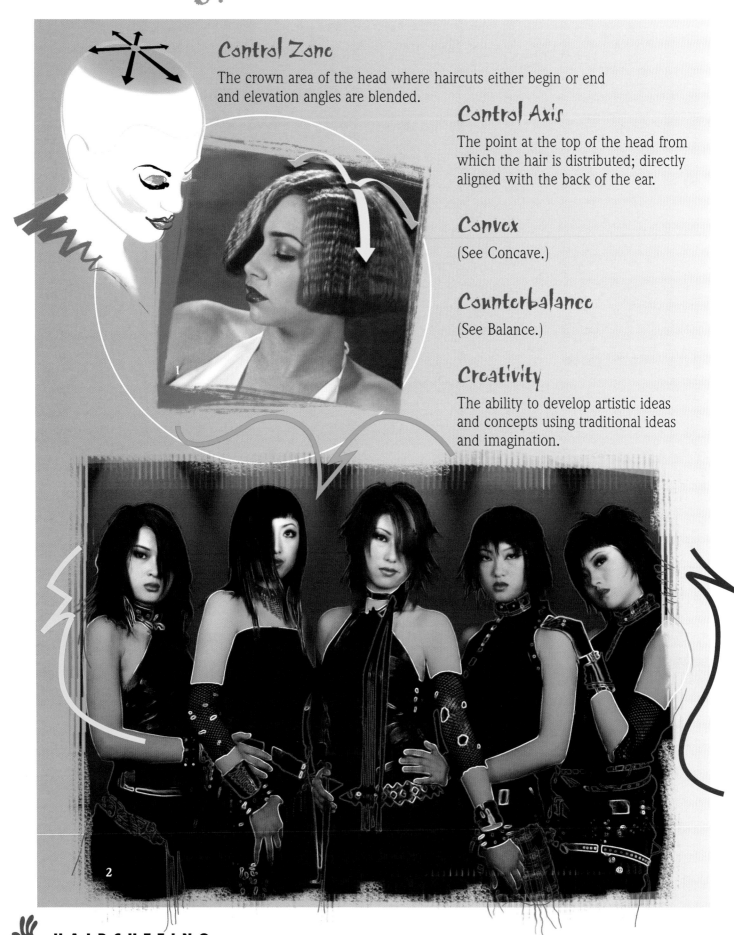

Control Zone

The crown area of the head where haircuts either begin or end and elevation angles are blended.

Control Axis

The point at the top of the head from which the hair is distributed; directly aligned with the back of the ear.

Convex

(See Concave.)

Counterbalance

(See Balance.)

Creativity

The ability to develop artistic ideas and concepts using traditional ideas and imagination.

1

2

Terminology

Cutting Techniques:

Elevation

An angle within the range from 0 degrees to 180 degrees created when the hair is lifted out from the head before being cut.

Shift

To move the hair from its natural growth direction to a different position when cutting.

Squeeze Cutting

A technique that compresses, or squeezes, the hair into a common area before it is cut.

Stacking

To graduate the hair using low elevation; the edges within the graduation create a bevel effect for volume and fullness.

Tension

The pulling of wet hair to stretch it before cutting.

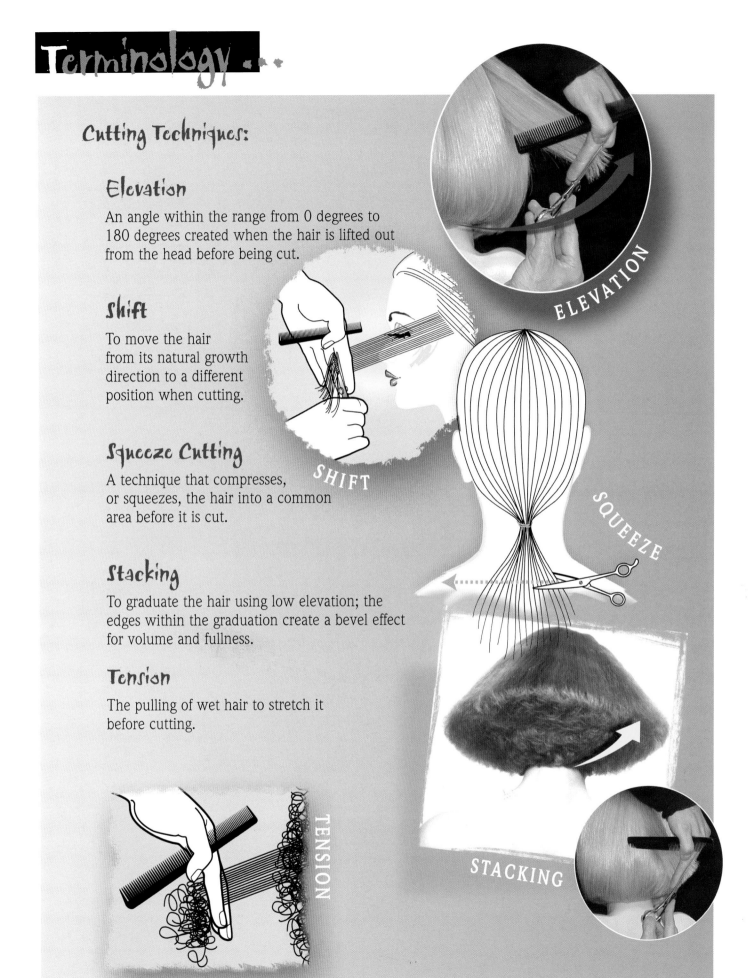

ELEVATION

SHIFT

SQUEEZE

STACKING

TENSION

Terminology...

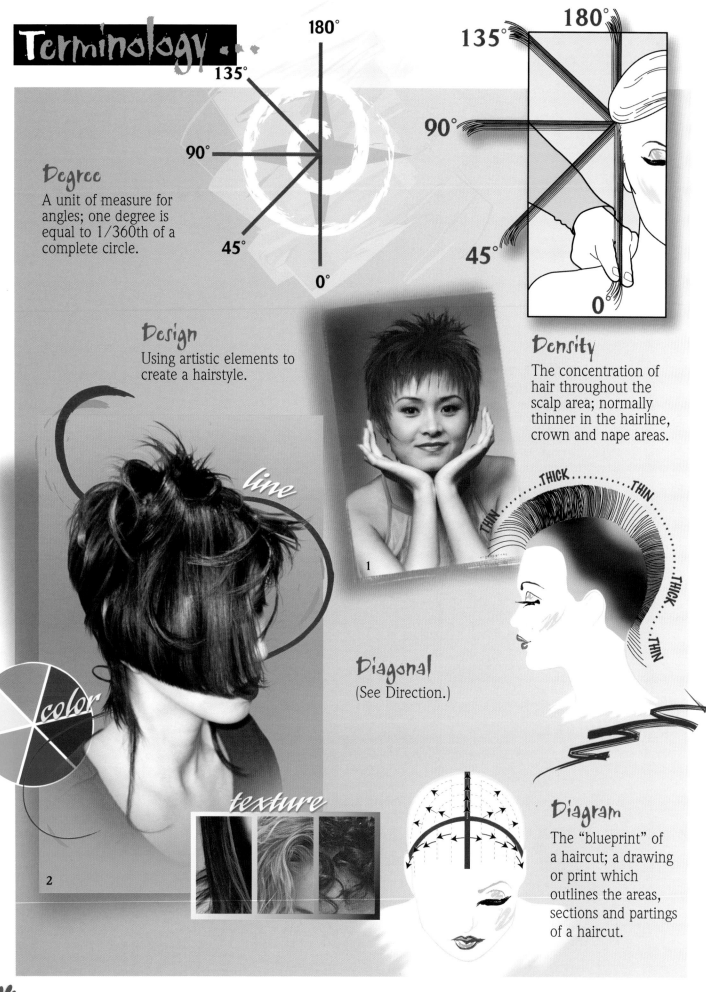

Degree
A unit of measure for angles; one degree is equal to 1/360th of a complete circle.

180°
135°
90°
45°
0°

180°
135°
90°
45°
0°

Design
Using artistic elements to create a hairstyle.

line

color

Density
The concentration of hair throughout the scalp area; normally thinner in the hairline, crown and nape areas.

THICK · · · · · · · · · · THIN
THIN
THICK
THIN

1

Diagonal
(See Direction.)

texture

2

Diagram
The "blueprint" of a haircut; a drawing or print which outlines the areas, sections and partings of a haircut.

Terminology

Dimension

A measurement of one or more directions. An unfinished haircut has two dimensions: length and width. Most finished hairstyles have three dimensions: length, width and depth.

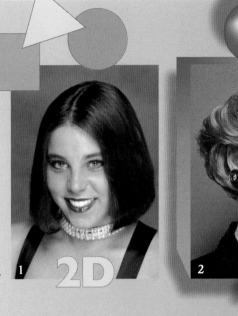

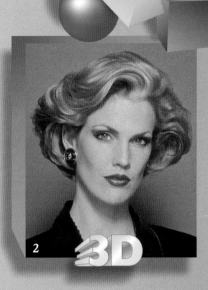

Direction:

Diagonal

A slanted or oblique line or plane.

Horizontal

A line or plane that is parallel to the earth's horizon; opposite of vertical.

Vertical

A line or plane extending up and down; opposite of horizontal.

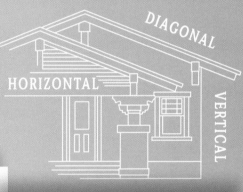

DIAGONAL
HORIZONTAL
VERTICAL

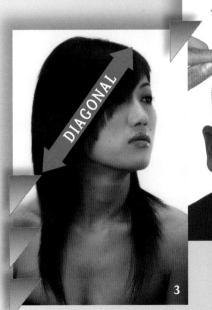

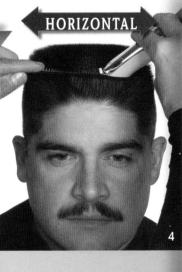

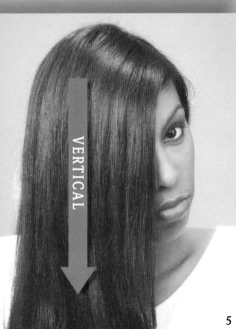

Terminology...

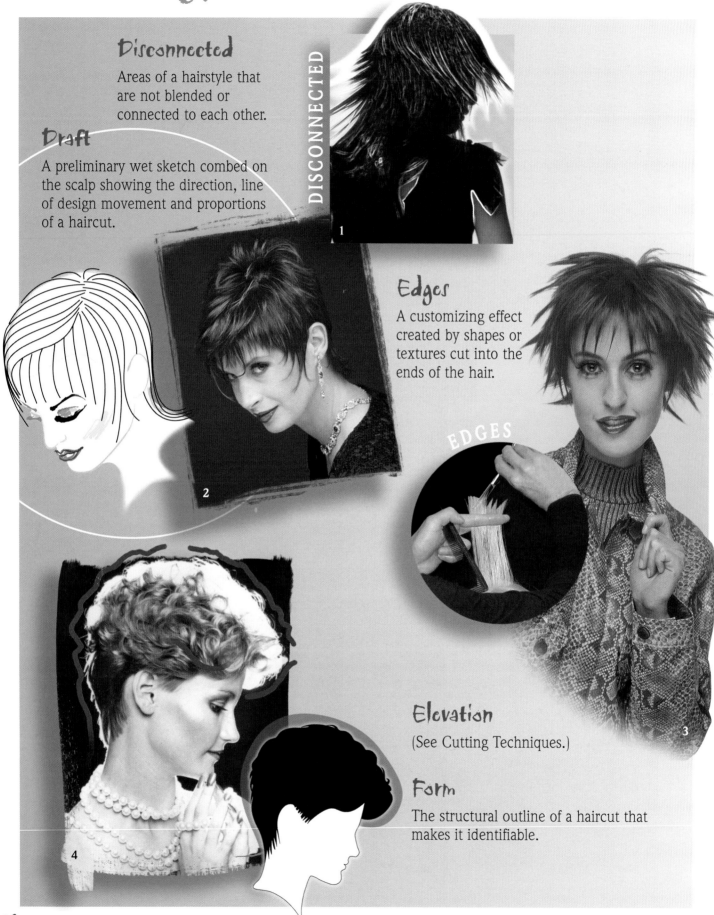

Disconnected

Areas of a hairstyle that are not blended or connected to each other.

DISCONNECTED

1

Draft

A preliminary wet sketch combed on the scalp showing the direction, line of design movement and proportions of a haircut.

2

Edges

A customizing effect created by shapes or textures cut into the ends of the hair.

EDGES

3

Elevation

(See Cutting Techniques.)

Form

The structural outline of a haircut that makes it identifiable.

4

Terminology

Free Stylin'
Cutting freehand with creativity and precision.

Functional Cuts
Haircuts suitable for the client's lifestyle.

Guides:

Stationary Guide
A fixed or non-moving guide used as a reference for the length of additional sections.

Traveling Guide
A guide that moves or passes from one section to another as a reference for the length of additional sections.

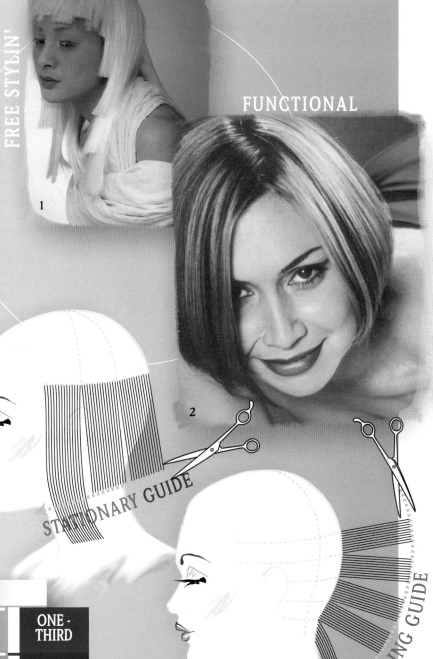

FREE STYLIN'

FUNCTIONAL

1

2

STATIONARY GUIDE

TRAVELING GUIDE

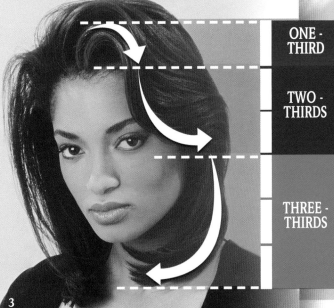

| ONE - THIRD |
| TWO - THIRDS |
| THREE - THIRDS |

3

Harmonic Progression
Arithmetic progression of sizes; the rhythmic movement of shapes, lengths and textures in a hairstyle, from smaller to larger and vice versa.

Terminology

Horizontal
(See Direction.)

Indentation Zone
(See Masses of the Head.)

Line
A border or boundary; the edge or division of a shape. Basic haircutting lines are vertical, horizontal and diagonal.

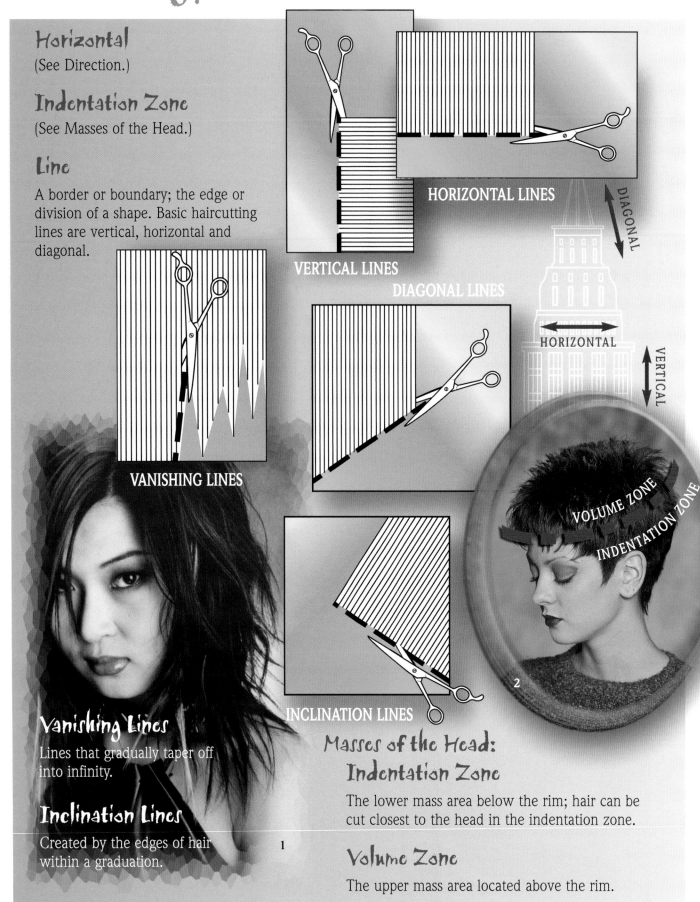

VERTICAL LINES

HORIZONTAL LINES

DIAGONAL LINES

DIAGONAL

HORIZONTAL

VERTICAL

VANISHING LINES

INCLINATION LINES

VOLUME ZONE

INDENTATION ZONE

2

Vanishing Lines
Lines that gradually taper off into infinity.

Inclination Lines
Created by the edges of hair within a graduation.

1

Masses of the Head:

Indentation Zone
The lower mass area below the rim; hair can be cut closest to the head in the indentation zone.

Volume Zone
The upper mass area located above the rim.

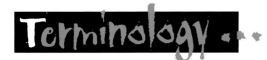
Terminology...

Neutral
Not possessing any particular quality; not negative or positive.

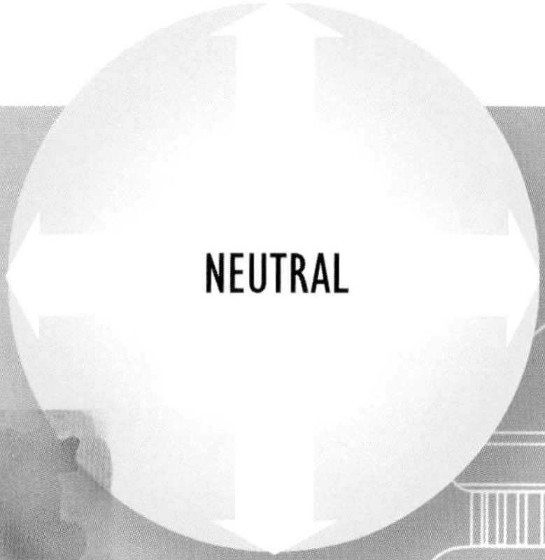

NEUTRAL

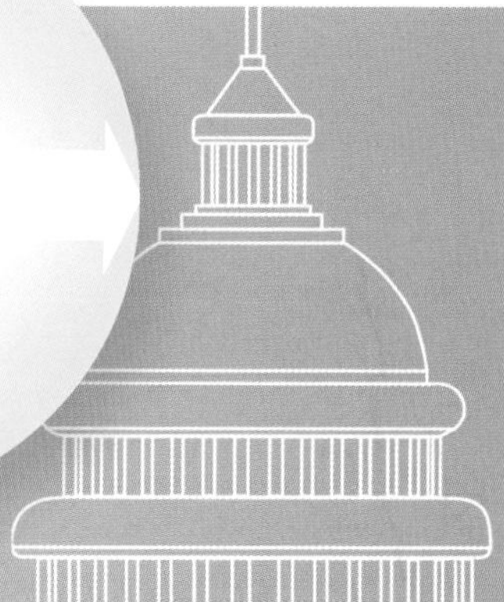

Order
An organized state, with elements logically coordinating with other groups of elements, all working harmoniously together.

Parallel
Lines and planes traveling in the same direction an equal distance apart.

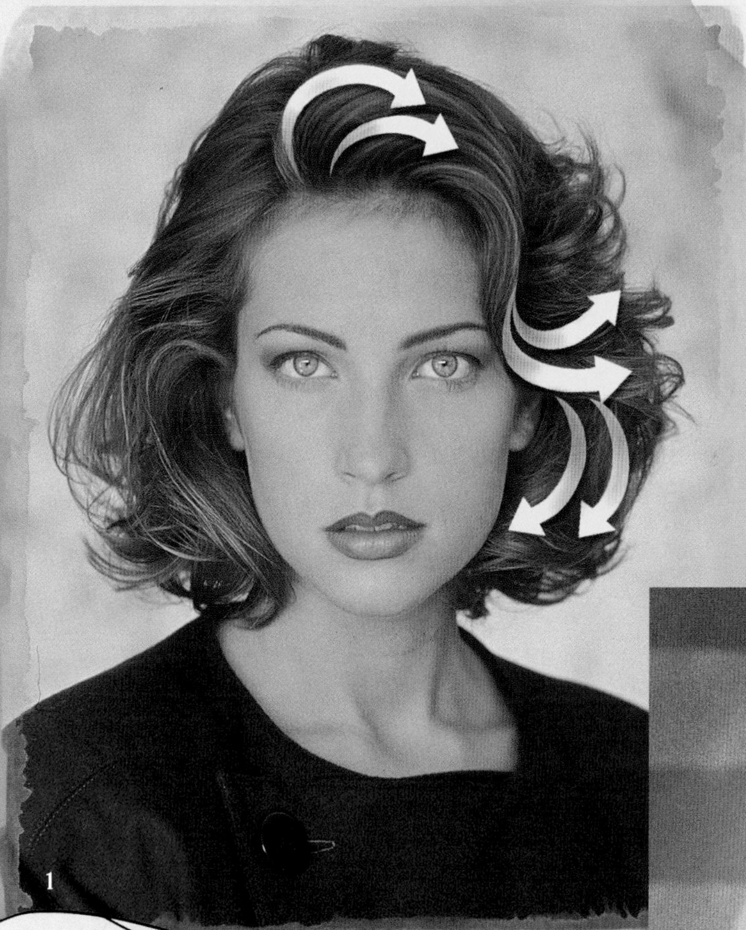

1

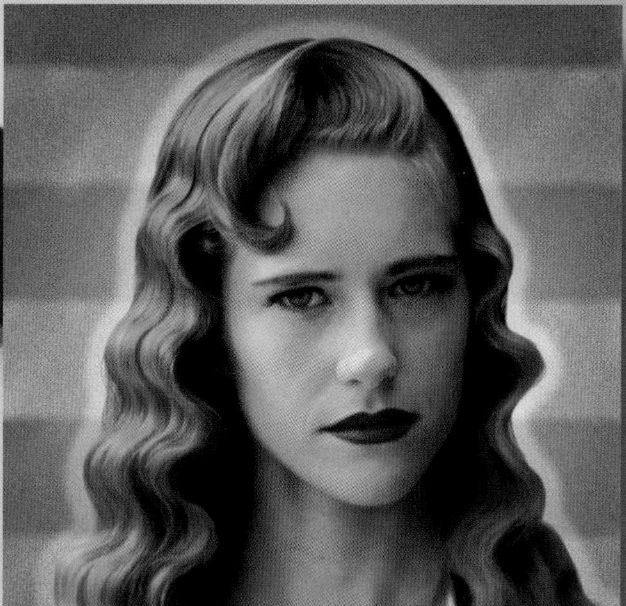

2

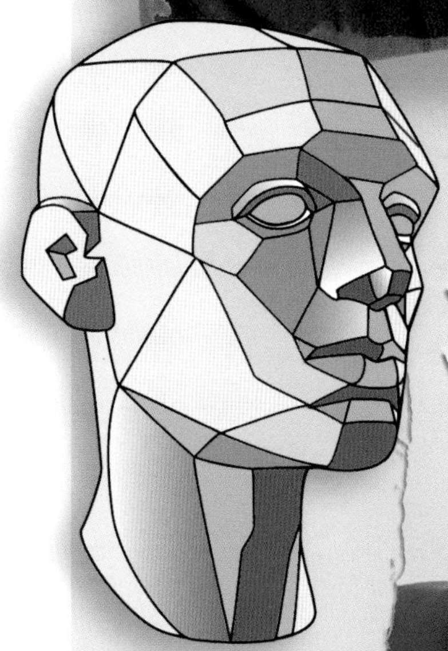

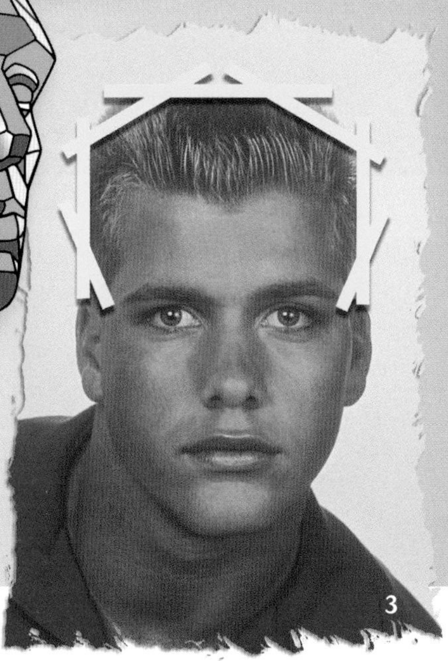

3

Plane
A flat or straight surface; a flat level area on a curved surface.

 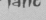

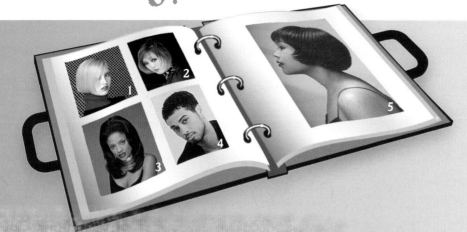

Portfolio

A case or folder for keeping photos or records of your hair creations.

Rim

The widest portion of the head where it curves; separates the volume zone from the indentation zone.

Salesmanship

The ability to sell by creating the need to buy a service or product.

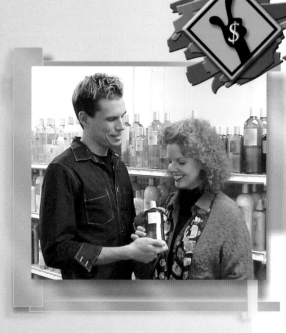

RIM

Shift Cutting

(See Cutting Techniques.)

Squeeze Cutting

(See Cutting Techniques.)

Stacking

(See Cutting Techniques.)

Stationary Guide

(See Guides.)

Tension

(See Cutting Techniques.)

Terminology...

Texture

The pattern, quality, feel and arrangement of individual hair strands within the overall hair structure; textures are described as fine, medium, coarse, straight, wavy and curly.

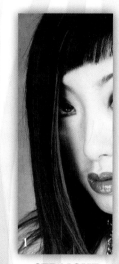
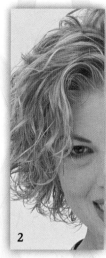
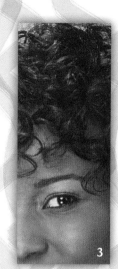

STRAIGHT   WAVY   CURLY

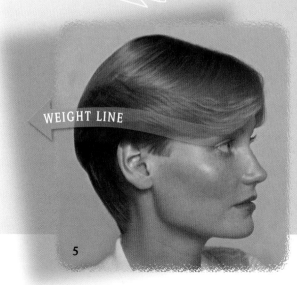

Theater

A room, space or area for demonstrating, teaching and presenting shows and other dramatic events.

Traveling Guide

(See Guides.)

Vertical

(See Direction.)

Volume Zone

(See Masses of the Head.)

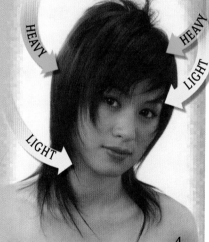

Weight

The concentration of hair within an area that gives the appearance of heaviness and density.

Weight Line

The line that separates low elevated hair from high elevated hair.

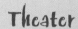

WEIGHT LINE

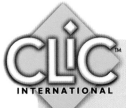

Haircutting Terminology REVIEW QUESTIONS

FILL IN THE BLANKS

✓ Abstract
✓ Balance
✓ Baseline
Concave
✓ Constructed
✓ Creativity
Dimension
✓ Disconnected
✓ Edges
✓ Free Stylin'
✓ Line
✓ Parallel
Salesmanship
Shift
Stationary
✓ Tension
Theater
Vanishing
✓ Vertical
✓ Weight Line

1. A harmonious arrangement of the elements of a hair design with nothing emphasized or out of proportion is in ___Balance___.

2. The line that separates low elevated hair from high elevated hair is called the ___Weight line___.

3. The ___Baseline___ is the outer boundary of a haircut.

4. A person with ___Creativity___ has the ability to develop artistic ideas and concepts using traditional ideas and imagination.

5. ___Tension___ is the pulling of wet hair to stretch it before cutting.

6. A measurement of one or more directions is called _____.

7. An ___Abstract___ design includes irregular shapes, colors or textures which maintain harmony within the overall form.

8. A ___Vertical___ line extends up and down.

9. Areas of a hairstyle that are not blended or connected to each other are ___Disconnected___.

10. ___Edges___ are a customizing effect created by shapes or textures cut into the ends of the hair.

11. A shape that curves inward is ___Concave___.

12. ___Salesmanship___ is the ability to sell by creating the need to buy a service or product.

13. Cutting freehand with creativity and precision is called ___Free Stylin___.

14. A _____ guide is a fixed or non-moving guide used as a reference for the length of additional sections.

15. To _____ the hair is to move it from its natural growth direction to a different position when cutting.

16. A border or boundary that creates the edge or division of a shape is called a ___Line___.

17. ___Parallel___ lines gradually taper off into infinity.

18. Lines and planes that travel in the same direction with an equal distance apart are _____.

19. A finished haircut with heavy ends and minimal action is called ___Constructed___.

20. A _____ is a room, space or area for demonstrating, teaching and presenting shows and other dramatic events.

STUDENT'S NAME   DATE   GRADE

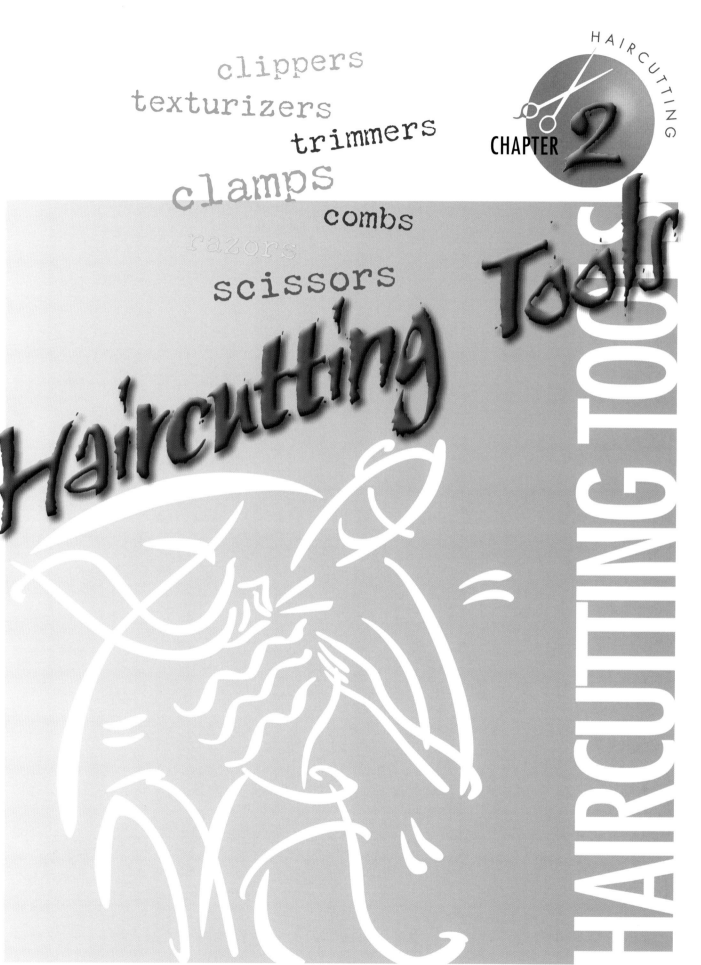

clippers

texturizers

trimmers

clamps

combs

razors

scissors

Haircutting Tools

Proper Haircutting Comb Usage

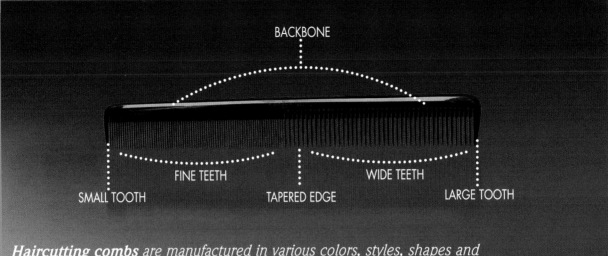

BACKBONE

FINE TEETH

SMALL TOOTH

TAPERED EDGE

WIDE TEETH

LARGE TOOTH

Haircutting combs are manufactured in various colors, styles, shapes and sizes. The combs are designed to help create the desired speed, taper and effects when cutting the hair.

Key elements of haircutting comb usage:

Placement: Placement of the comb in relationship to the hair will determine the angle and taper of the haircut. A good rule of thumb to remember is that the higher the angle of the comb, the shorter the hair will be cut.

Teeth: The wide teeth of the comb are used to detangle, distribute and part the hair. The fine teeth smooth the hair prior to cutting.

1) Distribute the hair with the wide teeth.

2) Use the fine teeth to create tension and smooth the hair.

3) Part the hair into sections with the wide tooth at the end of the comb.

Control: Practice the following comb control positions prior to cutting hair, so the tools will feel natural in your hands when you are ready to use them:

COMB AND TOOL COORDINATION: Learn to hold the comb and cutting tool (scissors or razor) together in your hands to eliminate the need to put the comb down while cutting. After the hair is parted and sectioned with the comb, hold the comb in your non-dominant hand between your thumb and index fingers. The comb may also be used to hold the ears down when cutting the hair around the ear area.

SCISSOR OVER COMB: The comb and scissors are used together, moving in sync with each other. The scissors should lay parallel and flat against the comb as it travels in an upward direction. The scissors are opened and closed very quickly as the comb travels to blend the cutting area without leaving marks in the hair.

CLIPPER OVER COMB: The clipper and comb work together to cut very close tapered effects. The comb can also be used to hold the hair at the desired angle for the clipper to travel across when cutting.

"Practice scissor over comb coordination against a wall, mirror or on a bald mannequin. Do not cut hair until you master the coordination needed to use the tools."

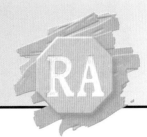

RA

Comb cleaning, disinfection and maintenance should be done on a regular basis in accordance with the appropriate regulatory guidelines.

Comb Dynamics ...

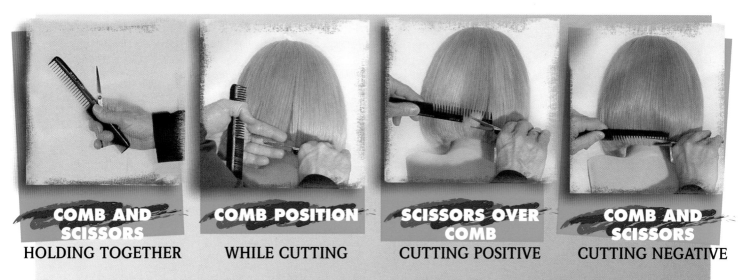

COMB AND SCISSORS
HOLDING TOGETHER

COMB POSITION
WHILE CUTTING

SCISSORS OVER COMB
CUTTING POSITIVE

COMB AND SCISSORS
CUTTING NEGATIVE

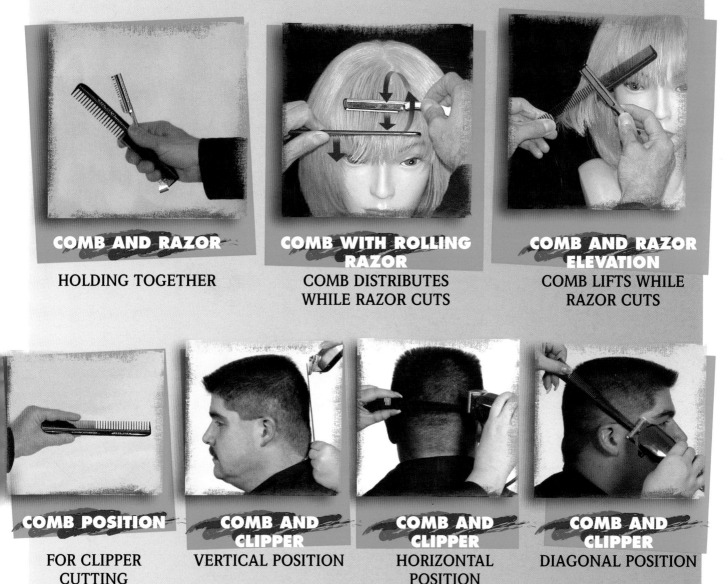

COMB AND RAZOR
HOLDING TOGETHER

COMB WITH ROLLING RAZOR
COMB DISTRIBUTES WHILE RAZOR CUTS

COMB AND RAZOR ELEVATION
COMB LIFTS WHILE RAZOR CUTS

COMB POSITION
FOR CLIPPER CUTTING

COMB AND CLIPPER
VERTICAL POSITION

COMB AND CLIPPER
HORIZONTAL POSITION

COMB AND CLIPPER
DIAGONAL POSITION

Cutting Combs ...

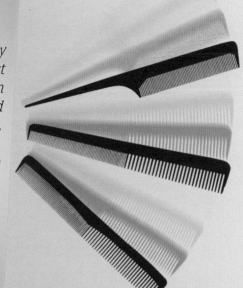

Like many tools a hairstylist owns, combs come in various styles and sizes, and have many functions. Styling, detangling, parting, sectioning, distributing and lacing are some of the ways you will use the following types of combs...

All-Purpose Cutting Comb

Perfect for use when cutting hair, the all-purpose comb is the most commonly used style. It is also a good choice to use when finger waving or clipper cutting hair.

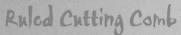

Ruled Cutting Comb

The ruled cutting comb is designed with measurements from 1" (2.5 cm) to 6" (15.2 cm) indicated on the backbone of the comb. These markings are used to measure the different hair lengths.

Rattail Comb

The rattail comb is used to distribute, shape and part the hair into sections. It is also used to weave strands for weave haircutting.

Tapered Hard Rubber Comb

Perfect for working close to the head, the tapered hard rubber comb has fine short teeth at one end and long coarse teeth at the other. It is also ideal for the scissors-over-comb technique.

Parting Comb

High-tech design and materials make the parting comb a favorite for precise parting and sectioning. The comb is designed for comfort, control and durability and is manufactured in a variety of sizes.

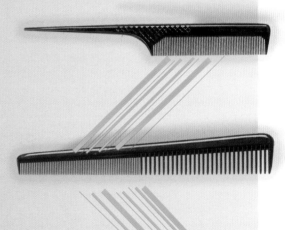

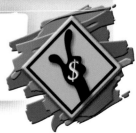

Professional combs help create professional results. A great retail item for the salon!

Texturizing Combs...

Jumbo Rattail Rake Comb

Texturizing combs help make haircut finishes exciting and there is a style for every texture. Each is designed to create a specific effect on the hair's surface. Following are only a few of the many varieties a hairstylist can use.

Specially designed with a long handle and widely-spaced teeth to comb deep lines and grooves into the hair.

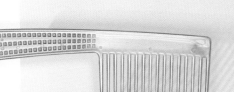

Rake Comb

The rake comb features teeth that are tapered to a point. This creates very wide spacing in the finished design. A great tool for curly hair to add lift, or for use when dry haircutting. Excellent tool for men's flat top haircuts.

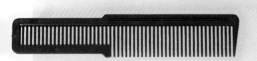

Clipper Comb

Clipper combs are specifically designed for use with clippers. The comb is constructed with long teeth that help clippers travel smoothly over the comb's surface, creating a more uniform cut. Excellent tool for men's flat top haircuts.

3-in-1 Comb

Texture, lift and lace all in one comb. The handle is constructed with five metal prongs for lifting and separating the hair strands.

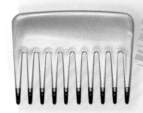

Finger Comb

The finger comb is designed to create a ruffled texture in short hair, and is especially suited for men's haircuts.

Curved Funnel Finger Comb

The shape and design of the teeth separate and funnel the hair; the curvature of the comb makes combing curved motion designs easier than using a straight comb.

Shark Tooth Comb

A great tool for short hair. The teeth separate the hair into deep pleats.

Proper Scissor Usage

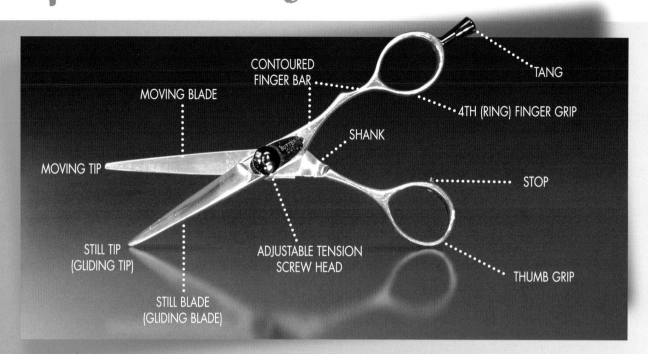

CONTOURED FINGER BAR

MOVING BLADE

TANG

4TH (RING) FINGER GRIP

SHANK

MOVING TIP

STOP

STILL TIP (GLIDING TIP)

ADJUSTABLE TENSION SCREW HEAD

THUMB GRIP

STILL BLADE (GLIDING BLADE)

Scissor Position:

When cutting, the scissors should remain parallel to the head, with the screw of the scissors facing outward. It is important to maintain proper control of the scissors to create high-precision haircuts.

Key elements of cutting with scissors:

Use only 1/3" (0.84 cm) to 1/2" (1.25 cm) of the scissor's cutting blade to cut the hair except when bulk cutting large amounts of hair (for example, speed cutting).

Never cut beyond the second knuckle of your middle finger. Cutting beyond this point will place the scissor past the straight, flat plane of the finger. This results in an increase in length when cutting palm facing scalp, and a decrease in length when cutting palm to palm.

Cut only with the moving blade. While the moving blade moves, the opposite blade (still blade) remains stationary. The thumb controls the moving blade. The still blade should not move up and down, but remain next to your fingers or the cutting surface on the outer perimeter of the head.

The angle of the cutting blade determines how the edges of the hair will turn and flow. This is referred to as **"putting English"** on the hair.

A scissor-over-comb technique is used to cut extremely short lengths of hair.

"Like a good artist has many brushes, you should collect a variety of scissors. They are a fundamental tool of haircutting."

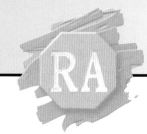

Cleaning and maintenance should be done on a regular basis. **See page 41.**

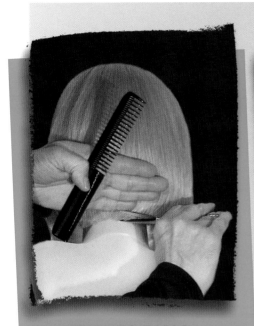

PALM TO PALM
0° LOW
HORIZONTAL ELEVATION
Cut on inside edge of finger.
Palm faces outward.

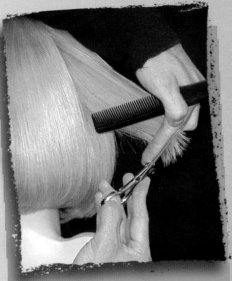

PALM TO SCALP
45° MEDIUM
VERTICAL ELEVATION
Cut on outside edge of finger.
Palm faces inward.

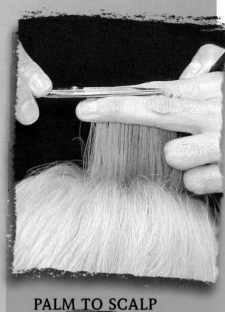

PALM TO SCALP
90°
VERTICAL ELEVATION
Cut on outside edge of finger.
Palm faces inward.

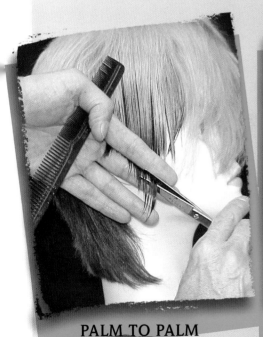

PALM TO PALM
0° LOW
DIAGONAL ELEVATION
Cut on inside edge of finger.
Palm faces outward.

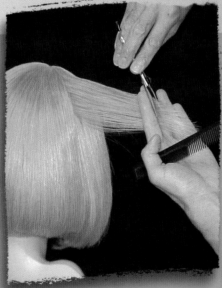

PALM TO PALM
45° REVERSE
VERTICAL ELEVATION
Cut on inside edge of finger.
Palm faces outward.

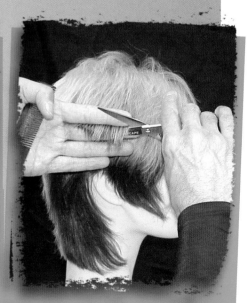

PALM TO PALM
90°
HORIZONTAL ELEVATION
Cut on inside edge of finger.
Palm faces outward.

Scissors

are a fundamental tool used in the art of cutting hair. Basic cuts with a large number of variations are used to create fashionable hair designs. A thorough knowledge of the many different types of scissors will help you create the styles you desire. Following are some examples of scissors you may use…

Standard Haircutting Scissors

The standard scissor is the most commonly used scissor and is manufactured in a variety of lengths. It holds hair firmly on the base of the blade and cuts evenly with very little pressure. High-quality standard scissors are generally designed with a tension control dial and hollow ground blades to hold and control hair for effortless results.

Blending Scissors

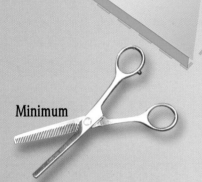

Minimum

Blending scissors are a type of tapering scissors commonly used to minimize bulk and create mobility in the cut. Unlike standard scissors, the moving blade has very fine, short teeth. The teeth are spaced 1/32" (0.8 mm) or less apart for minimum hair removal. Only the hair within the teeth is cut, creating a very fine taper to the hair. Blending scissors are manufactured in a variety of lengths.

Tapering Scissors

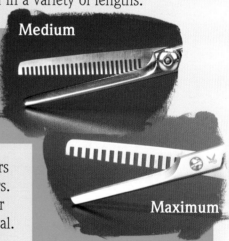

Medium

Maximum

Tapering scissors are available in various styles, and like the blending scissors, have one straight blade and one blade with teeth. The teeth are spaced close together on some styles and farther apart on others. The distance between the teeth determines the amount of hair that is cut and the degree of the taper. The teeth of tapering scissors are longer and cut deeper than those of the blending scissors. The teeth are spaced 1/16" (1.6 mm) apart for medium hair removal and 1/8" (3.2 mm) apart for maximum hair removal.

Weave Cut Scissors

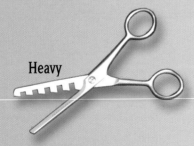

Heavy

Weave cut scissors are used to create layered, voluminous and wispy cuts. Irregular lengths and chunky edges can also be created. The still blade is smooth and the moving blade has notches spaced according to the texture desired. Weave cut scissors are manufactured in a variety of lengths and cutting blade designs.

Haircutting Scissors ...

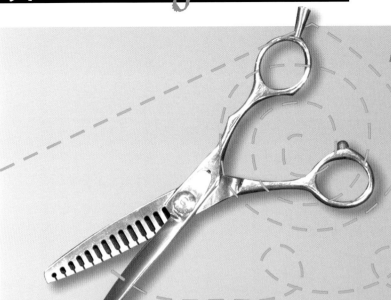

Motion Scissors

Motion scissors are specialized scissors that perform double duty. The stationary blade is smooth and hollow ground. The cutting blade has teeth that are designed to thin and notch with a tapered edge, giving motion to the hair.

Adjustable Scissors

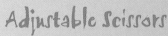

Advancements in cutting technology have created a scissor that can be adjusted to optimize your own personal comfort. Length, blade closure, and tension can be controlled as desired. The scissor adjusts from 4 1/2"(11.4 cm) to 5 1/2"(14 cm) in length. Adjustable scissors also feature a safety chain to prevent dropping.

Double Blade Thinning Scissors

Double blade thinning scissors have teeth on both sides; therefore, not all hair within the notches is cut. Single blade scissors will actually remove more hair than double blade scissors of the same size.

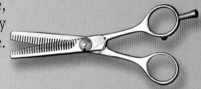

Cut and Tapering Scissors

The cut and tapering is a two-in-one scissor that cuts the outer strands of hair while tapering the inside strands.

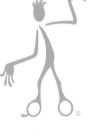

"Often in our industry, the words 'scissors' and 'shears' are used interchangeably. But for accuracy, only the word 'scissors' should be used to describe the haircutting tool. Let's examine the two Webster's Dictionary definitions."

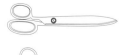

SHEARS – a pair of sharp cutting blades larger than, but similar to, those of a scissors, and often joined by a spring.

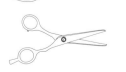

SCISSORS – a cutting tool consisting of two sharp-edged beveled blades which are pivoted near two handles through which finger and thumb are passed.

Tapering and Texture Scissors ...

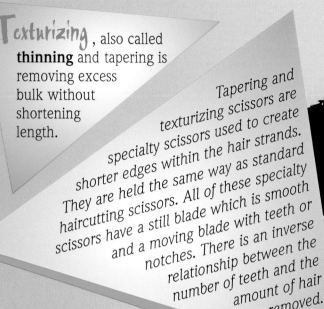

Texturizing, also called **thinning** and tapering is removing excess bulk without shortening length.

Tapering and texturizing scissors are specialty scissors used to create shorter edges within the hair strands. They are held the same way as standard haircutting scissors. All of these specialty scissors have a still blade which is smooth and a moving blade with teeth or notches. There is an inverse relationship between the number of teeth and the amount of hair removed.

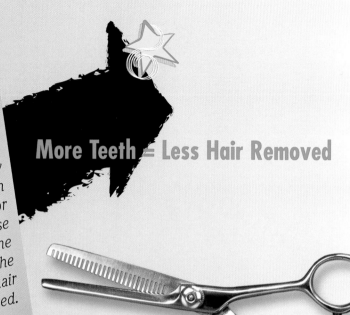

More Teeth = Less Hair Removed

The following table is a good reference guide for specialty scissors:

1/32" (0.8 mm) **TAPER OR BLENDING**		**MINIMUM** Hair Removal
1/16" (1.6 mm) TAPER		MEDIUM **Hair Removal**
1/8" (3.2 mm) **TAPER**		**MAXIMUM** Hair Removal
VARIOUS spacing of wide teeth : WEAVE CUT		HEAVY FRINGES **and extreme textures**

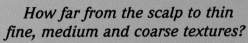

Tapering and Texture Scissors

How far from the scalp to thin fine, medium and coarse textures?

Fine: $\frac{1}{2}$ inch (1.25 cm)

Medium: 1 inch (2.5 cm)

Coarse: $1\frac{1}{2}$ inches (3.81 cm)

Texture

is created in hair by the notches, or teeth, in the cutting blade of the scissors. Variations in the spacing of the teeth, the depth of the teeth and the design of the cutting angles on the edges of the blades create the special effects that are cut into the hair strands.

Texturizing Scissors

There are many different texturizing scissors on the market. Weave cut, channel, notching and alpha are just a few of the types of texturizing scissors you may work with. The effect you wish to create will determine which texturizing scissor you use.

NOTE: Always place the texturizing scissors into the hair at the same angle as the cutting line on the outer or inner perimeter guideline.

"Always be 'a cut above the rest' by selecting the proper scissors for the cuts you perform!"

S.H.E.A.R.S.

6 Points of Purchasing Scissors ...

Steel

Consider the type of metal of which the scissors are made.
Most scissors contain iron, carbon and other alloys that provide strength and stainless properties. Scissors containing Molybdenum (Molly) Steel are flexible and less corrosive. Cobalt scissors are superior in strength and maintenance of a sharp edge. Also consider whether the scissors have been forged or cast. Forged scissors are more flexible and are generally of a higher quality than cast scissors. They are also more expensive.

By purchasing good scissors that are made of quality steel and fit your hand and cutting style comfortably, you invest in a lifetime tool for your professional career. The letters of the word SHEARS will help you remember the six key points of purchasing scissors.

Handle

There are generally two types of handles to choose from: straight and offset. Both handles are of even length in the straight style. In the offset style, one handle is slightly longer. This feature helps to reduce fatigue when cutting the proper way (with the thumb down). Personal comfort and cutting style will determine which type of handle is right for you.

Edge

Most scissors have beveled or convex edges. Beveled edges are more angular and are used to cut dry hair. Convex edges are shaped like the outside of a sphere and are used to cut wet hair or for slide cutting. Convex edges produce a smoother cut than beveled edges. It is important to know the difference between the two types of edges, not only when purchasing but also when inspecting the edges after sharpening. A nice convex edge given to the wrong sharpener can come back as a beveled edge. Hollow ground scissors hold a sharp cutting edge, which helps hold the hair while cutting through the strands.

Alignment

Alignment refers to the curve of the set of the blade. A properly aligned blade will be perfectly curved and meet at one spot all the way down the blade. A scissor that is out of alignment might "drag" in one place, therefore going dull and skipping over the hair without cutting it. Whether or not a scissor can be re-aligned depends on how it was formed. A cast scissor is impossible to align because its brittleness will cause it to break if bent. However, cast scissors rarely become misaligned. Forged scissors are easier to align because they are more flexible and can be bent back into position.

Ride Line

The ride line (also called the tracking line) is the silver line along the edge of the scissor. The presence of this line indicates a scissor of high quality. The line should be shiny and smooth with no stripes crossing through it. A ride line with stripes indicates that the scissor was finished on a machine. The best scissors are hand-honed on a Japanese wet stone. Remember to test the pair of scissors prior to purchase. Every scissor is different and testing a sample pair of scissors gives you a true feel for how the scissors cut.

Source

The source is where you buy your scissors. It is a good idea to purchase scissors from someone who is knowledgeable about the scissors they sell and who is capable of maintaining your scissors for you. Be certain that you know and trust the supplier, because the different types of steel cannot always be distinguished by visual inspection alone.

C.L.A.S.S.

Scissors Care and Maintenance ...

Cleaning

Clean your scissors between every haircut. When the blades of scissors are covered with hair, moisture and chemicals, rust can occur. Regular cleaning also keeps the blades sharp longer.

- Remove dirt and build-up. Use a chamois or soft cloth to wipe the blades.
- Disinfect the blades. Use rubbing alcohol or an oil-based clipper disinfectant. Do not use a water-based disinfectant, because it will corrode the blades.
- Clean underneath the screw head. Use a piece of dental floss to remove debris without taking the scissors apart.

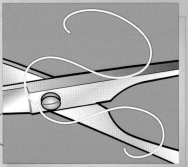

In any profession, the proper care and maintenance of tools is important. As a hairstylist, scissors are a critical tool and can be an expensive investment. The letters of the word CLASS will help you remember the key elements of caring for your scissors for peak performance.

Lubrication

Lubricate your scissors at the end of each day. A coating of oil will protect the screw by sealing out moisture. It will also keep the scissors feeling smooth. Use scissor oil or sewing machine oil for lubrication. Clipper oil is not recommended because of its thickness.

- Scissors with adjustable screws—oil between the blades and on the back side of the screw head.
- Scissors with flat screws—oil the screw head and between the blades.

Adjustment

Adjust your scissors after lubricating them, or when they fold hair instead of cutting it. Proper scissor adjustment is often a matter of personal preference. However, a good rule of thumb is that when the scissors are held open with the blades at right angles to each other in the shape of a cross, the handle that is dropped will swing freely without dropping so far as to touch the other handle. Scissors are adjusted in one of two ways:

- Scissors with adjustable screw heads—turn pin right to tighten, left to loosen. Remember, righty-tighty and lefty-loosey.
- Scissors with screws—imagine the screw head as the face of a clock. Using a screwdriver, turn the screw five minutes on the face of a clock. Check the scissors and adjust more if needed. Do not turn more than five minutes at a time to prevent over-adjusting.

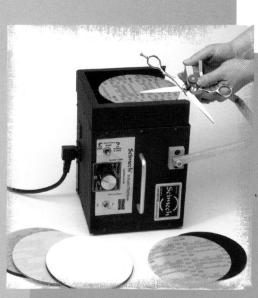

Storage

Store your scissors in a safe container at all times when not in use. Never put your scissors in an unprotected area where curious children can reach them. Instead, secure and store them in a stand or case where they stay safe and dry.

Sharpening

Sharpening your scissors will either extend their life...or shorten it! Most scissors require sharpening every three to six months. Always take your scissors to a reputable sharpener who is trained to work on haircutting scissors. An inexperienced sharpener or one without the right equipment could destroy your scissors.

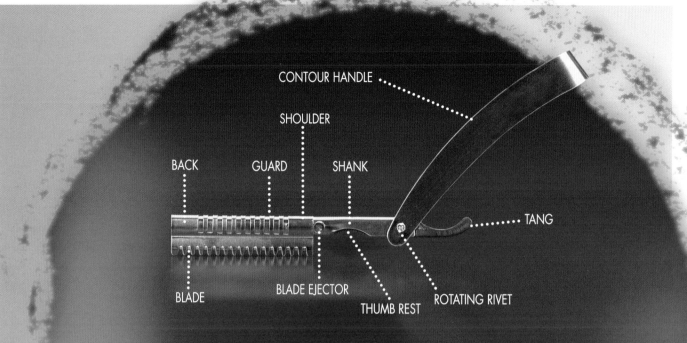

CONTOUR HANDLE

SHOULDER

BACK   GUARD   SHANK

TANG

BLADE   BLADE EJECTOR   ROTATING RIVET

THUMB REST

Correct Razor Position:

Correct razor position is important when razor cutting. The guard always faces the stylist and the razor blade faces the hair. The specific razor technique used determines the amount of pressure applied, and ultimately the amount of hair that is removed.

Razor cutting *is performed with a* *continuous stroking* *action* *that creates soft, light and wispy ends. The proper stroking action and angle of the blade determines the amount of hair removed.*

Razor texturizing is used to customize haircuts. Always examine each client's natural texture, growth direction and thickness of hair prior to razor texturizing to determine how to best create the desired effects.

Key guidelines for razor cutting:

When razor cutting, **the hair should always be wet,** except when texturizing very curly hair.

The angle of the blade influences the amount of hair that is removed. A good rule of thumb: when holding the razor, the number of fingers on top of the razor will determine the amount of pressure used when cutting.

Always use a sharp blade to prevent pulling the hair. NEVER use a rusty razor blade, which could cause infection if the skin is accidentally cut.

Use caution to **avoid cutting moles, scars or any skin lesions.**

Use a guard on your razor for protection, whenever applicable. Never put a razor in your pocket. Reaching for the razor could cause serious injury.

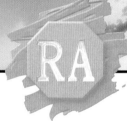

Follow appropriate local regulatory guidelines for sanitation and disinfection of disposable razors and blades. Always discard razors and blades in a container with a lid, for safety.

Razor Dynamics ...

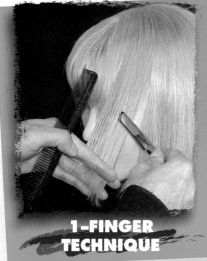

1-FINGER TECHNIQUE

MINIMUM PRESSURE
One finger creates minimum pressure, flexibility and the least amount of hair removal.

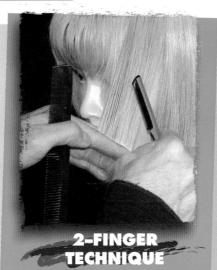

2-FINGER TECHNIQUE

MEDIUM PRESSURE
Two fingers provide medium pressure when cutting and removing hair.

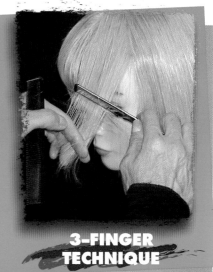

3-FINGER TECHNIQUE

MAXIMUM PRESSURE
Three fingers give maximum control and maximum hair removal.

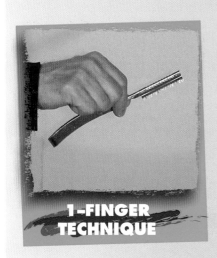

1-FINGER TECHNIQUE

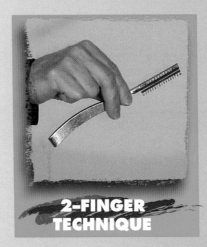

2-FINGER TECHNIQUE

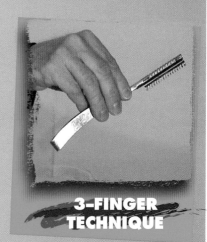

3-FINGER TECHNIQUE

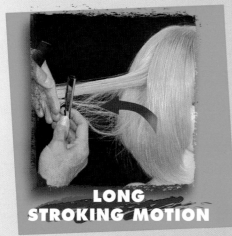

LONG STROKING MOTION

Produces soft, wispy taper to hair strands and ends.

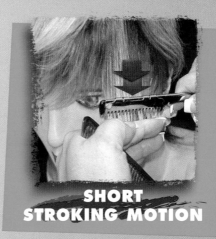

SHORT STROKING MOTION

Produces soft and light lines or jagged edges.

Haircutting Razors

A **razor** *can be used to create a special tapered effect on the edges of the hair strand. There are many different types of razors, each designed to create various hairstyles. As you develop your own style, you'll decide which razors are best for you!*

All-Purpose Hair Shaping Razor

As the name implies, the all-purpose razor has many uses, including haircutting, tapering or shaving. One type of all-purpose razor is the safety razor, which features a removable safety guard and a single-edge replaceable razor blade.

Shaping Razor

The shaping razor is designed to cut and create special effects on the hair strands. It is typically used to cut tapered, layered, beveled, blunt, concave or convex haircuts.

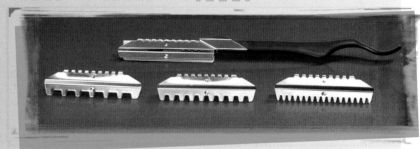

Fingertip Razor

Worn on the tips of the fingers, the fingertip razor is used for tapering and to form special effects on the hair shaft and ends of the hair.

Texturizing Razor

The texturizing razor is used for texturizing and special effects cutting. It utilizes a replaceable double-head blade with adjustable texturizing attachments for creative razor cutting.

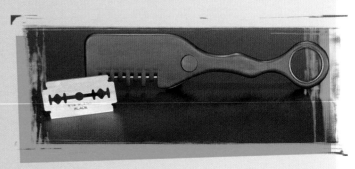

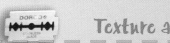

Texture and Taper Razor

Like the texturizing razor, the texture and taper razor does not cut in a straight line. One side of the razor creates a fine taper, and the opposite side cuts like a weave cut scissor. The texture and taper razor has double-head notches, a comfort fit handle and uses double-head razor blades. This razor is available in one- or two-blade designs, in plastic or metal form.

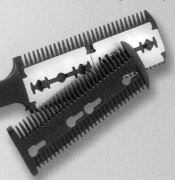

Disposable Razor Trimmer

This inexpensive disposable razor is designed to cut with precision. Caution: the blade is very sharp and has no guard. This razor is perfect for texturizing, special effects, and making precise cuts in hard-to-reach areas.

Texturizing Cutting Comb

The unique design of the texturizing cutting comb allows for a razor blade to be placed inside one-half of the comb. This enables you to texturize or cut the hair using a comb-like tool.

"Always be sure to use a sharp razor for your cuts. Use caution when changing razor blades, so you don't cut yourself!"

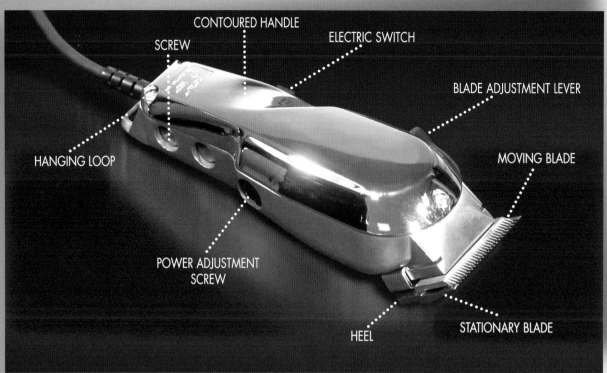

CONTOURED HANDLE
SCREW
ELECTRIC SWITCH
BLADE ADJUSTMENT LEVER
HANGING LOOP
MOVING BLADE
POWER ADJUSTMENT SCREW
HEEL
STATIONARY BLADE

Clipper Position:

Practice the upward arching position against a bald mannequin. This will help you develop coordination and flexibility in your wrist prior to cutting actual hair.

Key elements of clipper cutting:

Hold the clipper lightly to allow flexibility in the wrist.

An **upward arching position,** in which the heel is against the head with the blades facing upward into the hair, **is used to create the various degrees of elevation** within a cut.

A **downward inverted position,** in which the heel is facing away from the head and the blade points directly into the hair, **is used for clean, precise lines**.

To cut the hair, the blades of the clipper move either **horizontally** across the hair from the outside to the inside, **vertically** in an upward or downward movement, or **diagonally** in a slanted line.

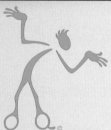

"The clipper is a versatile tool that is used to cut extremely short lengths and also for the removal of large quantities of hair in one cut."

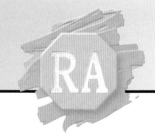

RA

Cleaning, disinfection and maintenance should be done on a regular basis in accordance with appropriate regulatory guidelines. *See page 49.*

Clipper Dynamics

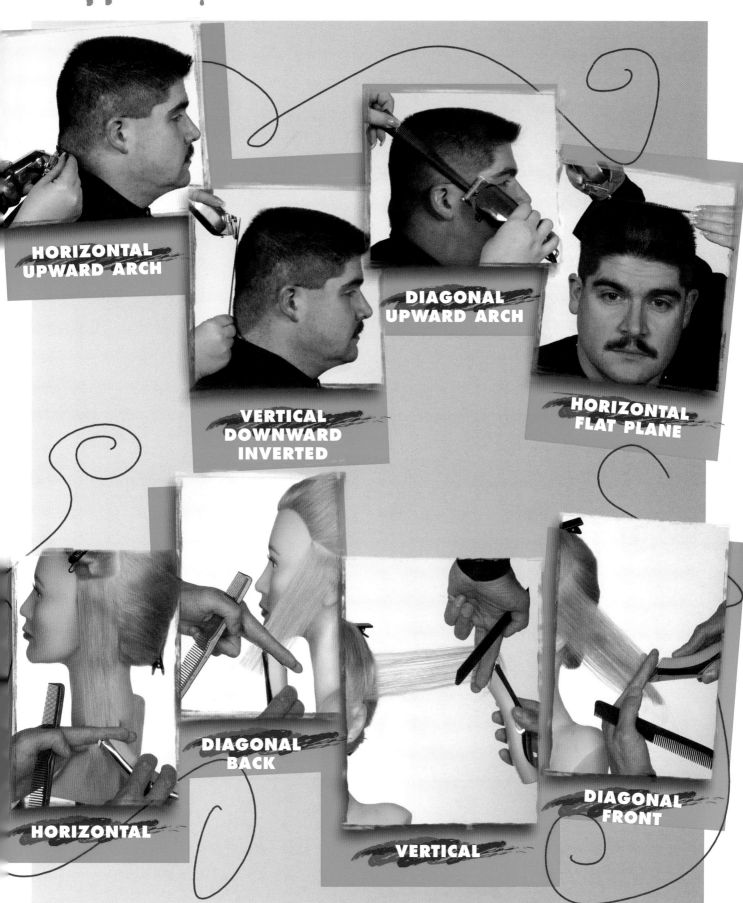

HORIZONTAL UPWARD ARCH

VERTICAL DOWNWARD INVERTED

DIAGONAL UPWARD ARCH

HORIZONTAL FLAT PLANE

HORIZONTAL

DIAGONAL BACK

VERTICAL

DIAGONAL FRONT

Clippers and Trimmers ...

Electric Clippers Plus Attachments

Electric clippers are used to cut, fade, taper, trim, thin, feather, channel and fringe a haircut. Various attachments (guards) are available, which allow you to cut the hair to a specific length. Clippers are a great tool for creating flat top and crew cut styles.

Although clippers and trimmers can be used to cut an entire head of hair, they are often used for creating special effects within a cut. The following tools are used to give customized looks to hair, beards and mustaches...

T-Blade Trimmer Plus Attachments

T-blade trimmers are used to trim close to the head, and to give line definition to the outer perimeter of the hair. They are especially helpful for trimming around the ears.

Outline Trimmer

The outline trimmer is used primarily for beard trimming, hair art and outer perimeter design work. The lightweight, cordless, rechargeable design makes it perfect for quick touch-ups.

Clippers and Trimmers ...

Sideburn, Ear and Nose Trimmer

This handy battery-operated trimmer cleans up all of those hard-to-reach areas. It makes a great retail item.

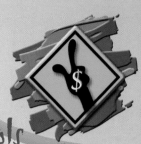

Clipper Maintenance Tools

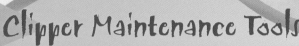

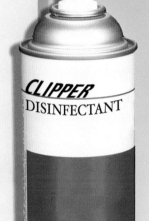

Clipper Disinfectant

A germicide made especially for clippers, this spray is an easy and fast way to sterilize your clipper. Apply before using clippers on a client.

Clipper Oil

Using clipper oil will keep your clippers running smoothly by protecting and lubricating the moving blades. Just add a drop or two of oil after brushing out the clipper head and cutting blade.

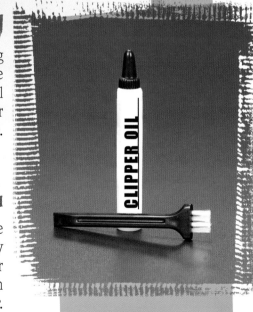

Clipper Cleaning Brush

This miniature brush is specially designed to get into all of the small spaces of the clipper head and blades to remove stray pieces of hair. Be sure to thoroughly clean your clipper with the brush prior to oiling it, to prevent the oil and hair from building up and clogging your clipper.

Proper Airformer Usage...

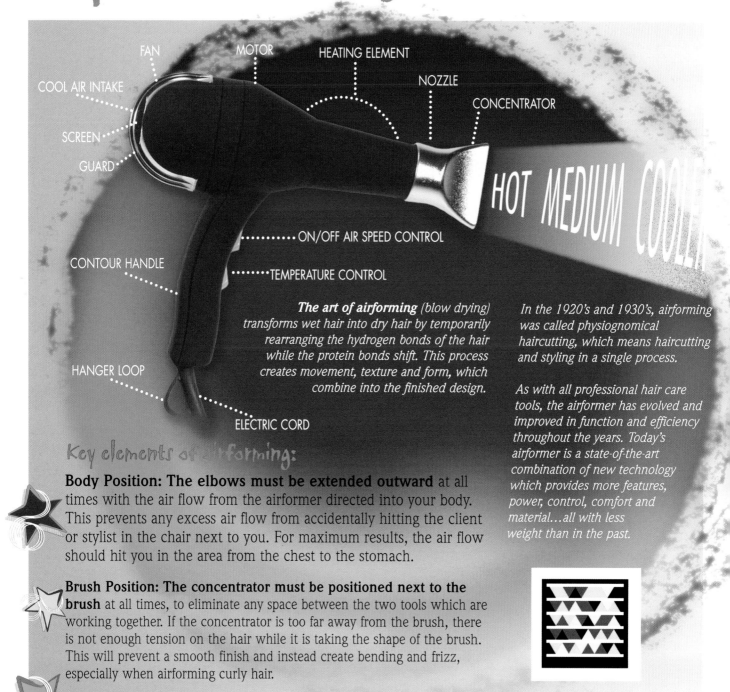

FAN
MOTOR
HEATING ELEMENT
NOZZLE
CONCENTRATOR
COOL AIR INTAKE
SCREEN
GUARD
ON/OFF AIR SPEED CONTROL
CONTOUR HANDLE
TEMPERATURE CONTROL
HANGER LOOP
ELECTRIC CORD

HOT MEDIUM COOL

The art of airforming (blow drying) *transforms wet hair into dry hair by temporarily rearranging the hydrogen bonds of the hair while the protein bonds shift. This process creates movement, texture and form, which combine into the finished design.*

In the 1920's and 1930's, airforming was called physiognomical haircutting, which means haircutting and styling in a single process.

As with all professional hair care tools, the airformer has evolved and improved in function and efficiency throughout the years. Today's airformer is a state-of-the-art combination of new technology which provides more features, power, control, comfort and material...all with less weight than in the past.

Key elements of airforming:

Body Position: The elbows must be extended outward at all times with the air flow from the airformer directed into your body. This prevents any excess air flow from accidentally hitting the client or stylist in the chair next to you. For maximum results, the air flow should hit you in the area from the chest to the stomach.

Brush Position: The concentrator must be positioned next to the brush at all times, to eliminate any space between the two tools which are working together. If the concentrator is too far away from the brush, there is not enough tension on the hair while it is taking the shape of the brush. This will prevent a smooth finish and instead create bending and frizz, especially when airforming curly hair.

Air Flow Direction: Begin by distributing the hair into the desired direction until 50 percent of the water is removed. **Position the brush to work with the air flow** to create the hair movement in the desired direction. Rotate the brush until the hair is completely dry. **Never shake the airformer from side to side,** which creates fuzzy hair strands. Instead, learn to polish the hair by rotating the brush in the same direction as the cuticle whenever possible.

Set The Curl: After the hair is dry, **set the curl by heating the base of the brush then letting it cool** to set the hair in position. Do not remove the brush until the hair is cool, or it will lose its form. Use a rocking motion with alternating heating and cooling.

"For a more in-depth study of European airforming techniques, please refer to the CLiC Hairdesigning Module."

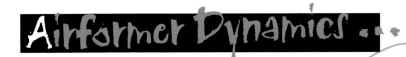

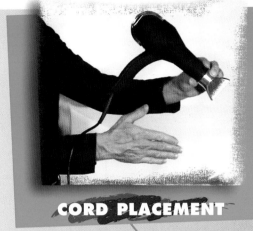

CORD PLACEMENT

Place over arm for maximum control.

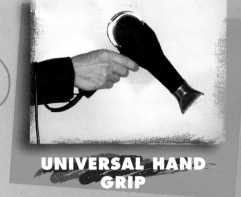

UNIVERSAL HAND GRIP

Always grip handle.
Never grip nozzle.

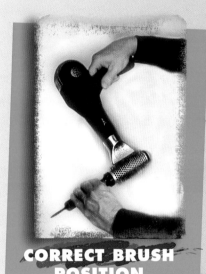

CORRECT BRUSH POSITION

Keep concentrator directly
next to brush.

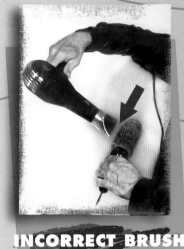

INCORRECT BRUSH POSITION

Eliminate any space between
concentrator and brush.

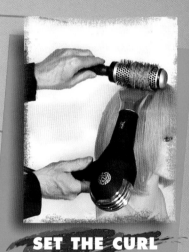

SET THE CURL

Use tension to straighten.
Relax tension to curl.

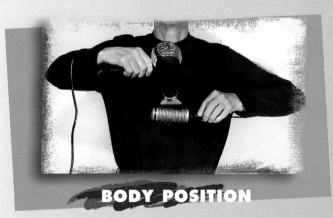

BODY POSITION

Extend the elbows outward. Direct airflow inward.

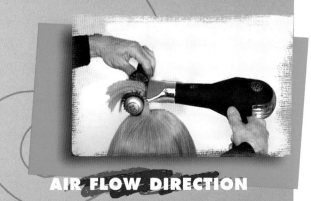

AIR FLOW DIRECTION

Follow the natural direction of the cuticle.

Airformers and Attachments ...

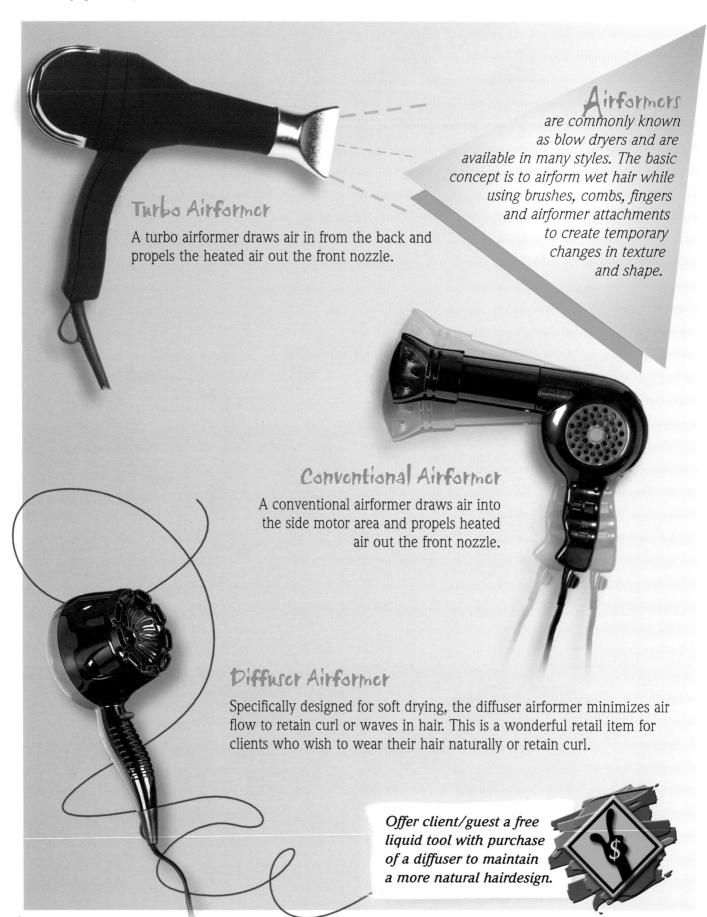

Airformers
are commonly known as blow dryers and are available in many styles. The basic concept is to airform wet hair while using brushes, combs, fingers and airformer attachments to create temporary changes in texture and shape.

Turbo Airformer

A turbo airformer draws air in from the back and propels the heated air out the front nozzle.

Conventional Airformer

A conventional airformer draws air into the side motor area and propels heated air out the front nozzle.

Diffuser Airformer

Specifically designed for soft drying, the diffuser airformer minimizes air flow to retain curl or waves in hair. This is a wonderful retail item for clients who wish to wear their hair naturally or retain curl.

Offer client/guest a free liquid tool with purchase of a diffuser to maintain a more natural hairdesign.

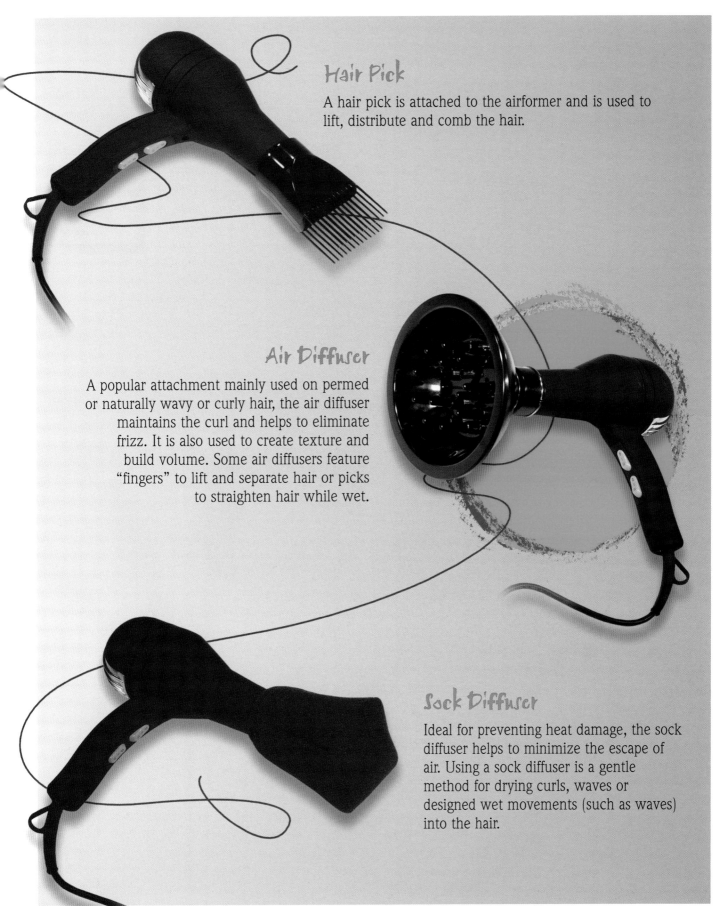

Hair Pick

A hair pick is attached to the airformer and is used to lift, distribute and comb the hair.

Air Diffuser

A popular attachment mainly used on permed or naturally wavy or curly hair, the air diffuser maintains the curl and helps to eliminate frizz. It is also used to create texture and build volume. Some air diffusers feature "fingers" to lift and separate hair or picks to straighten hair while wet.

Sock Diffuser

Ideal for preventing heat damage, the sock diffuser helps to minimize the escape of air. Using a sock diffuser is a gentle method for drying curls, waves or designed wet movements (such as waves) into the hair.

Airforming Brushes...

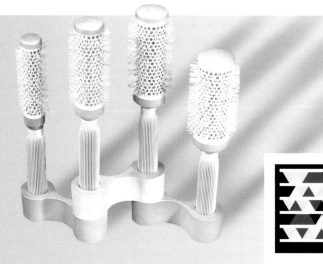

Your choice of styling brush will determine the quality of your finished style. Brushes are available for many different functions, such as to help curl hair, shorten drying time, prevent split ends and polish hair to a healthy sheen. The desired effect will determine the type of brush you will use to create your masterpiece.

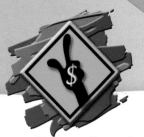

The use of high quality professional brushes helps clients maintain their haircuts. Teach your clients how to properly use brushes, so they will want to purchase them for at home use!

Thermal Metal Round Brush

Designed with short, synthetic, heat-resistant bristles, the thermal metal round brush features an aerated metal barrel that retains heat from the airformer, causing hair to curl faster. The effect is similar to hot rollers and curling irons. Some brush styles feature a removable pin in the handle that provides parting precision. This brush can be used on all hair lengths and is available in a variety of barrel sizes.

Plastic Round Brush

The plastic round brush is used with an airformer to add texture and curl to hair. Constructed with plastic, rubber or wood handles and short, synthetic, heat-resistant bristles, the brush is also available with beaded tips to prevent scalp abrasion. This brush can be used on most hair lengths and is available in a variety of barrel sizes.

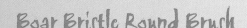

Boar Bristle Round Brush

The boar bristle round brush works similar to a curling iron when forming hair around the metal base of the brush during airforming. The brush is made of natural boar bristles, which are softer than most synthetic bristles. Because they don't cut into the hair when brushing, boar bristles help polish the hair and prevent split ends. The brush is available in a variety of diameters and some styles feature a retractable pin in the handle base.

Airforming Brushes . . .

Porcupine Round Brush

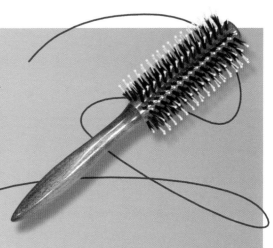

The porcupine round brush contains a combination of synthetic and boar hair bristles. The synthetic bristles grip the hair, then help to detangle and distribute it into the brush. The boar bristles smooth and polish the hair to help prevent tangling and split ends. The brush is available in oval or rectangular shapes.

Pin Type Brush

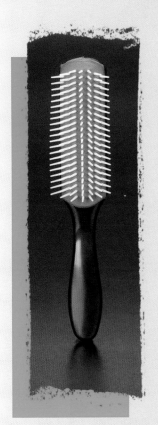

Used for smoothing, shaping and polishing hair, the pin type brush is constructed of heat-resistant synthetic materials. It is designed with up to 9 rows of replaceable bristles and can be used on all types and lengths of hair. The rubber-based back helps eliminate static electricity when used with an airformer.

Double Back Vent Brush

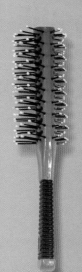

The double back vent brush features short, widely spaced bristles on one side for root lifting and volume, and longer bristles on the other side for hair distribution. Some styles have beaded bristles that help prevent split ends and scalp abrasion. The brush design enables quick hair drying time when working with airformers.

Cushioned Wire Vent Brush

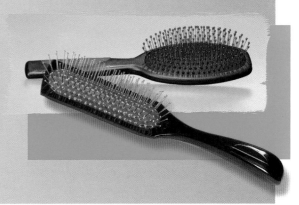

Constructed with wire bristles and beaded plastic tips to prevent scalp abrasion, the cushioned wire brush is used to relax sets, brush out tangles before shampooing and remove tangles after shampooing. The rubber base of the brush helps to eliminate static electricity when used on dry hair. It is available in a variety of shapes and sizes and should NOT be used for airforming.

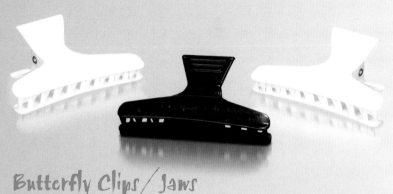

Clips
are used to secure hair and are available in many different variations. Popular styles include butterfly, marcel, duckbills and wave comb clamps.

Butterfly Clips / Jaws

Butterfly clips, or jaws, are designed to secure large sections of hair. They are manufactured in a variety of colors.

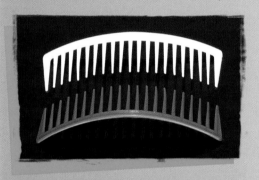

Wave Combs

Designed to fit the shape of the head, the curved wave combs interlock and are made of flexible, lightweight plastic. An excellent choice to hold a wave formation or to secure a wave formation into wet hair when free stylin'. Wave combs are also good for securing hair when dry haircutting.

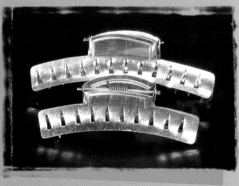

Marcel Clamps

Marcel clamps are designed to create strong ridge waves, and may also be used like a butterfly clamp for a strong hold. Manufactured in lightweight aluminum.

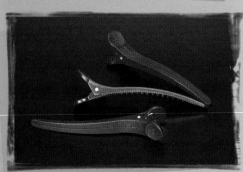

Duckbill Clips

Duckbills are designed to secure the hair for sectioning, parting and twisting the hair prior to cutting. They are available in plastic or aluminum, and in a variety of colors and lengths.

Cutting Accessories

Shown here are just a few of the many products that will aid you in creating your haircutting masterpieces.

Spray Bottle

Available in every shape and color imaginable, the spray bottle dispenses water in a controlled fashion.

Waist Tool Pouch

The waist tool pouch offers an easy way to keep your tools within reach and provides an excellent way to keep them organized.

Cutting Collar

The cutting collar rests flat on the back of the cape, creating a firm cutting surface. Some collars are available with pre-marked curved or straight cutting guides. The collar also protects the covered area from chemical exposure.

Hand Mirror

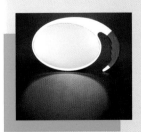

Show off that great cut! Let your client see every aspect of your haircutting skill. A large professional hand mirror allows your clients to view their haircuts at 360°.

Liquid Tools ...

There are many types of liquid cutting and styling tools on the market today. Following are just a few product examples...

Setting Lotion

Setting lotion is used when curling, blow drying and roller setting a style. This non-flaking, non-sticky solution provides protection against heat and is available in a variety of holding powers.

Glaze

Glaze can be used as a finishing lotion for roller setting, airforming and iron curling. It adds body and shine to a finished style and helps to control frizzy hair.

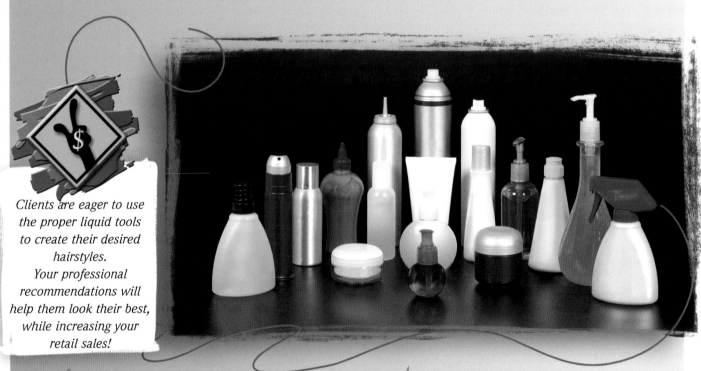

*Clients are eager to use the proper liquid tools to create their desired hairstyles.
Your professional recommendations will help them look their best, while increasing your retail sales!*

Gel

Gel also acts as finishing lotion, but offers more holding power than glazing lotions. Gel adds body to the hair and creates a firm hold when dried.

Mousse

Mousse gives hair definition and adds ample control, volume and shine.

Detangler

A detangler is used to smooth and detangle hair. It adds shine to the style without adding volume.

Finishing Spray

Finishing spray is used to hold a style in place. Finishing sprays are available in many hold strengths, from light hold to super freeze hold.

Smoothing Lotion

Smoothing lotion usually comes in a cream-type liquid and is applied to wet hair to help control curls, waves or damaged ends.

Liquid Tools ...

Pomade

Pomade is available in a variety of strengths and consistencies. Its uses vary. Some pomades can be used on both the scalp and hair; others are used strictly for styling to add shine and separation to the hair. Pomades with a heavy consistency cause the hair strands to stick together, resulting in maximum separation and texture.

Oil

Formulated to produce shine, separation and texture control, oils also help smooth the hair strands for manageability and softness. Oils are available in liquid, gel or spray formulas and light, medium or heavy consistencies.

Styling Wax

Remember the 5 "S"s of professional styling waxes: water-Soluble, Shine, Separation, Strength and Smoothness.

Thermal Spray

Thermal spray protects the hair from heat when using airformers, curling irons or hot rollers. A thermal barrier is sprayed onto the hair prior to applying heat. The heat activates protective elements that also add body to the hair.

Cutting Lotion

Cutting lotion is sprayed onto the hair prior to cutting. It helps smooth the hair for friction-free cutting. Cutting lotions are also great for slide and special effects cutting.

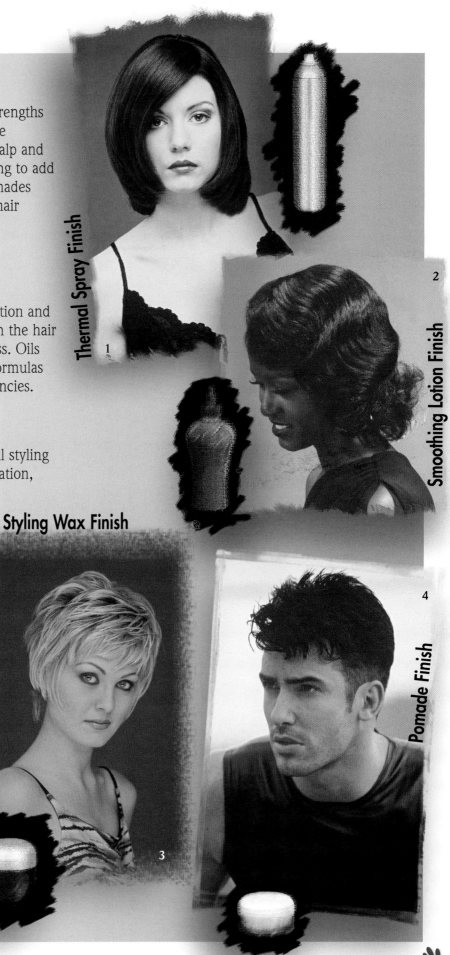

Thermal Spray Finish

1

Smoothing Lotion Finish

2

Styling Wax Finish

3

Pomade Finish

4

Computer Tools ...

We are living in the "information age" and it touches the professional salon industry just like all the other industries. The salon computer is rapidly becoming one of the most important tools for the hairstylist. It helps organize and prioritize the work load, and stores accurate client records, dates and services provided.

Try going online for educational and professional information, ordering products or finding out about trade shows. Network with your peers by visiting chat rooms that focus on the cosmetology industry. You can exchange ideas about cuts and styles, and gain valuable information about what's hot for the upcoming fashion season.

Software

Proper software is the key to managing a salon. It can run the front desk, organize payroll and keep client records current.

Compact Discs

A fun way to learn at your own pace!

Internet Access

A great way to research all aspects about the cosmetology field and stay informed about current and upcoming trends.

Computer Imaging System

This special computer is designed to allow clients to see new hair designs before their hair is touched. Haircuts, color and perms can be previewed to ensure that the client is happy with the results.

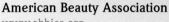

The internet is an exciting tool that helps bring people together from across the world to share ideas, information and friendship. It continues to grow in popularity and scope. This page is just a sample of the "world of information" about the cosmetology industry, waiting at your fingertips!

American Beauty Association
www.abbies.org

Beauty Net
www.beautynet.com

Beauty Professionals Networking on the Net
www.beautytech.com

Beauty Walk
www.beautywalk.com

Behind the Chair – MAN I CAN!
www.behindthechair.com
Certified Learning in Cosmetology®
www.clicusa.com

For Girls with Curls
www.naturallycurly.com

Hair Boutique
www.hairboutique.com

Hairfashion Portal
www.hairfinder.com

Hair Styles
www.hair-styles.org
Hair Today
www.hairtoday.com

National Cosmetology Association®
www.salonprofessionals.org

SalonBiz®
www.salonbiz.com

Professional Beauty Association
• **AACS** American Association of Cosmetology Schools
• **CEA** Cosmetology Educators of America
• **TSA** The Salon Association
   www.probeauty.org

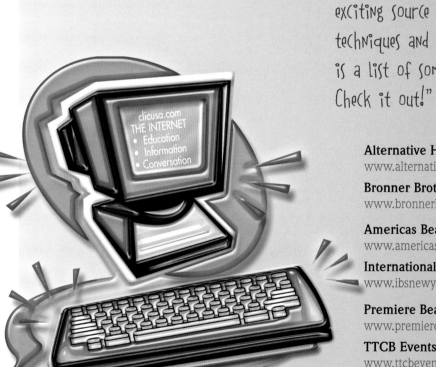

"You are on a journey of lifelong learning in the field of cosmetology. Professional hair shows are an exciting source for the latest trends, fashions, techniques and education in the industry. Following is a list of some of the biggest shows in America. Check it out!"

Alternative Hair Show
www.alternativehair.org

Bronner Brothers Atlanta Hair Show
www.bronnerbros.com

Americas Beauty Show (Chicago Midwest Beauty Show)
www.americasbeautyshow.com

International Beauty Show – New York, NY
www.ibsnewyork.com

Premiere Beauty Show Group
www.premiereshows.com

TTCB Events – Beauty Show Management
www.ttcbevents.com

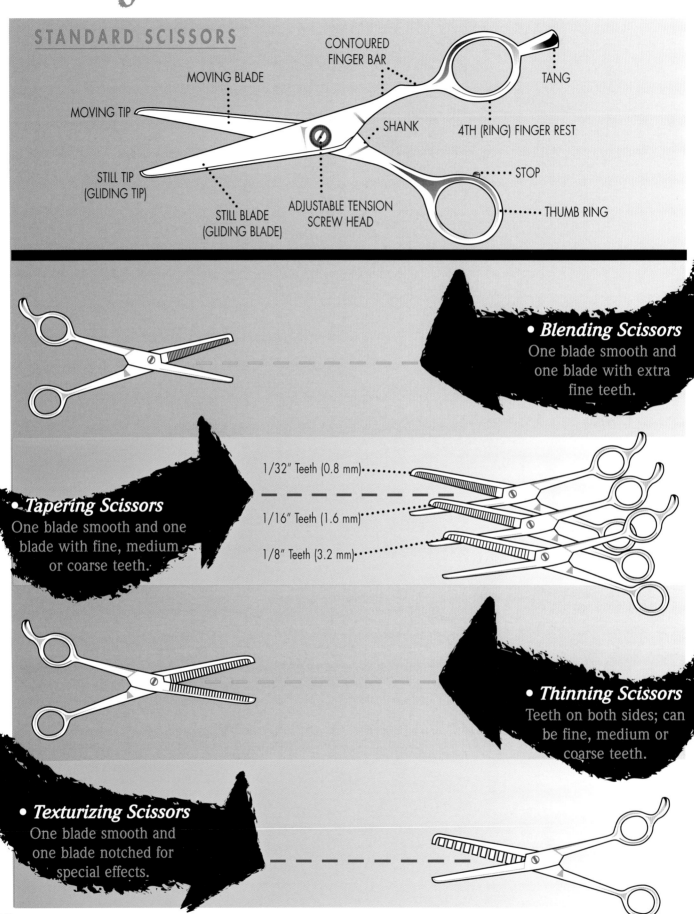

STANDARD SCISSORS

CONTOURED FINGER BAR

MOVING BLADE

TANG

MOVING TIP

SHANK

4TH (RING) FINGER REST

STILL TIP (GLIDING TIP)

STOP

STILL BLADE (GLIDING BLADE)

ADJUSTABLE TENSION SCREW HEAD

THUMB RING

• **Blending Scissors**
One blade smooth and one blade with extra fine teeth.

• **Tapering Scissors**
One blade smooth and one blade with fine, medium or coarse teeth.

1/32" Teeth (0.8 mm)

1/16" Teeth (1.6 mm)

1/8" Teeth (3.2 mm)

• **Thinning Scissors**
Teeth on both sides; can be fine, medium or coarse teeth.

• **Texturizing Scissors**
One blade smooth and one blade notched for special effects.

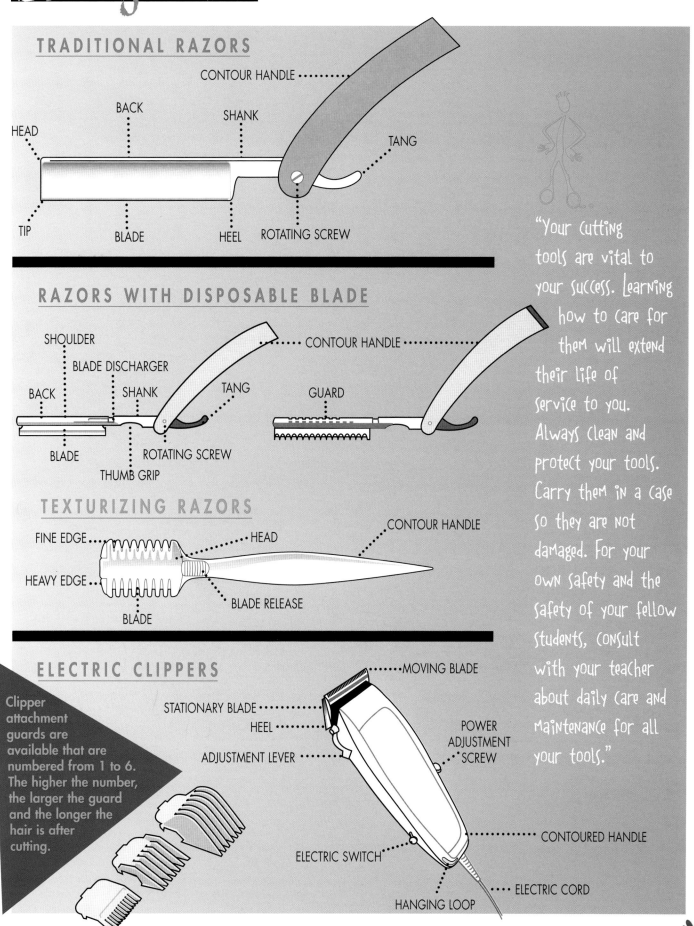

TRADITIONAL RAZORS

CONTOUR HANDLE

BACK

SHANK

HEAD

TANG

TIP

BLADE

HEEL

ROTATING SCREW

RAZORS WITH DISPOSABLE BLADE

SHOULDER

BLADE DISCHARGER

CONTOUR HANDLE

BACK

SHANK

TANG

GUARD

BLADE

ROTATING SCREW

THUMB GRIP

TEXTURIZING RAZORS

CONTOUR HANDLE

FINE EDGE

HEAD

HEAVY EDGE

BLADE RELEASE

BLADE

ELECTRIC CLIPPERS

MOVING BLADE

STATIONARY BLADE

HEEL

POWER
ADJUSTMENT
SCREW

ADJUSTMENT LEVER

Clipper attachment guards are available that are numbered from 1 to 6. The higher the number, the larger the guard and the longer the hair is after cutting.

CONTOURED HANDLE

ELECTRIC SWITCH

ELECTRIC CORD

HANGING LOOP

"Your cutting tools are vital to your success. Learning how to care for them will extend their life of service to you. Always clean and protect your tools. Carry them in a case so they are not damaged. For your own safety and the safety of your fellow students, consult with your teacher about daily care and maintenance for all your tools."

HOLDING THE SCISSORS

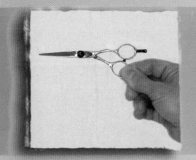

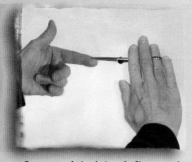

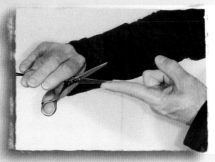

• Hold scissors with the screw head facing toward you.

• Insert 4th (ring) finger into the 4th finger grip. The grip should not pass your second knuckle.

• Place thumb into the thumb grip. Remaining fingers rest on top of the still blade.

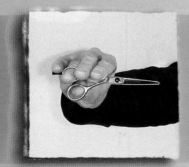

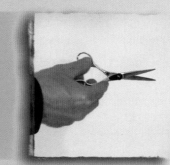

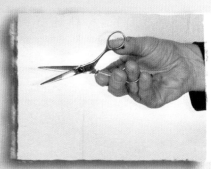

RECOMMENDED POSITION

Cutting toward yourself allows you to see the line develop. It also prevents the hair from being pushed as you close the scissors, resulting in a high precision cut.

ALTERNATE POSITION

Cutting away from yourself with the thumb up prevents you from seeing the line develop. The hair is lifted and pushed out the front of the scissors, decreasing the precision of the cut.

ERGONOMIC ALERT

Using the alternate position when cutting puts the hand and wrist in a twisted position which may cause discomfort and development of carpal tunnel syndrome.

EXERCISE

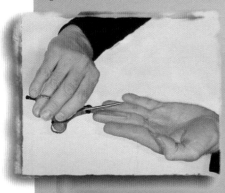

PALM TO PALM CUTTING

• Open the scissors using only your thumb.
• Do not cut beyond the second knuckle of your middle finger.
• Keep the still blade against your hand or the cutting surface on the client.

"Always keep your elbows out, and do not bend from the waist when cutting. This keeps your body in a straight line with your cut. Practice these important positions while practicing your cutting techniques."

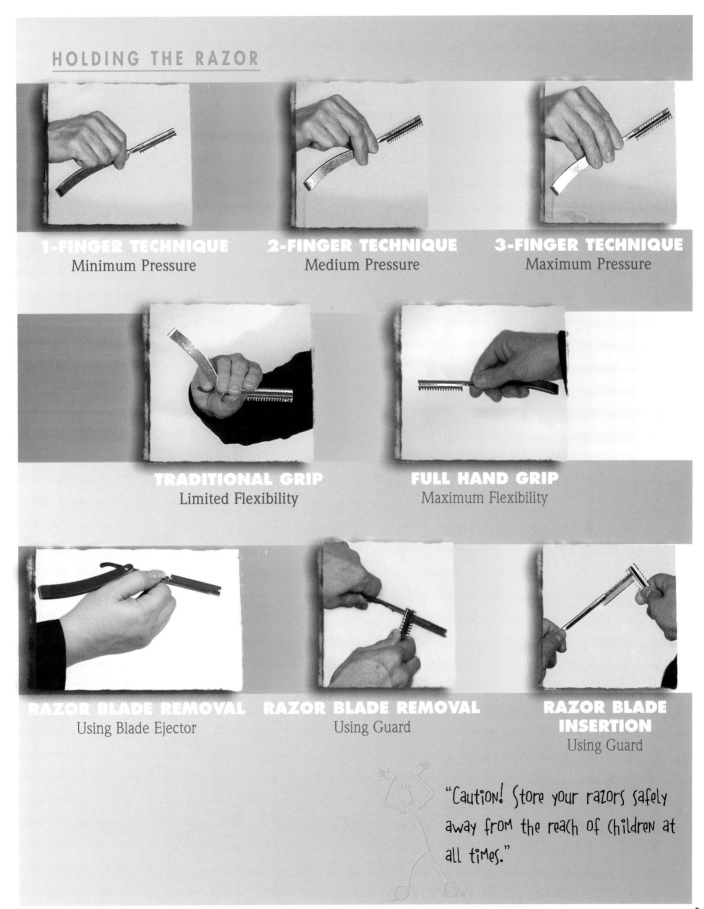

HOLDING THE RAZOR

1-FINGER TECHNIQUE
Minimum Pressure

2-FINGER TECHNIQUE
Medium Pressure

3-FINGER TECHNIQUE
Maximum Pressure

TRADITIONAL GRIP
Limited Flexibility

FULL HAND GRIP
Maximum Flexibility

RAZOR BLADE REMOVAL
Using Blade Ejector

RAZOR BLADE REMOVAL
Using Guard

RAZOR BLADE INSERTION
Using Guard

"Caution! Store your razors safely away from the reach of children at all times."

HOLDING THE CLIPPERS — CREATING THE ARCH

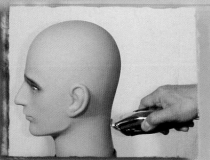 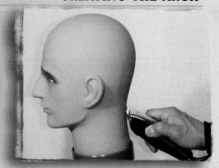 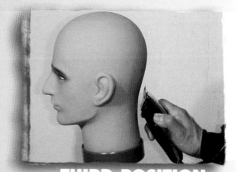

FIRST POSITION
Straight into line of cut

SECOND POSITION
Travel against neck

THIRD POSITION
Curve upward and outward

CUTTING PLANES OF THE HEAD — COMB PULLS HAIR TO ANGLE OF CUT

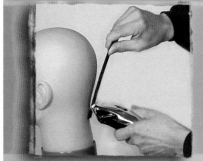 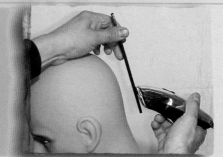 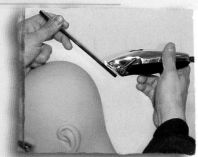

CENTRAL NAPE AREA

OCCIPITAL AREA

CROWN AREA

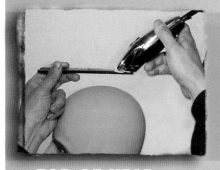 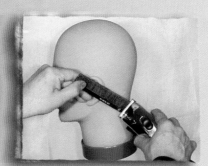 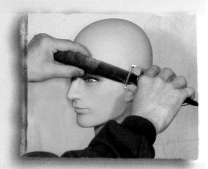

TOP OF HEAD

DIAGONAL NAPE

TEMPORAL AREA

OUTLINING THE EARS

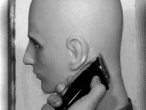 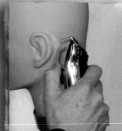 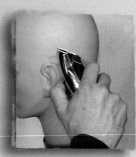 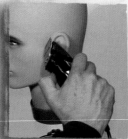 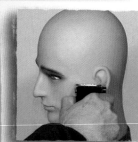

LOWER EAR **MIDDLE EAR** **UPPER EAR** **FRONT OF EAR** **SIDEBURN**

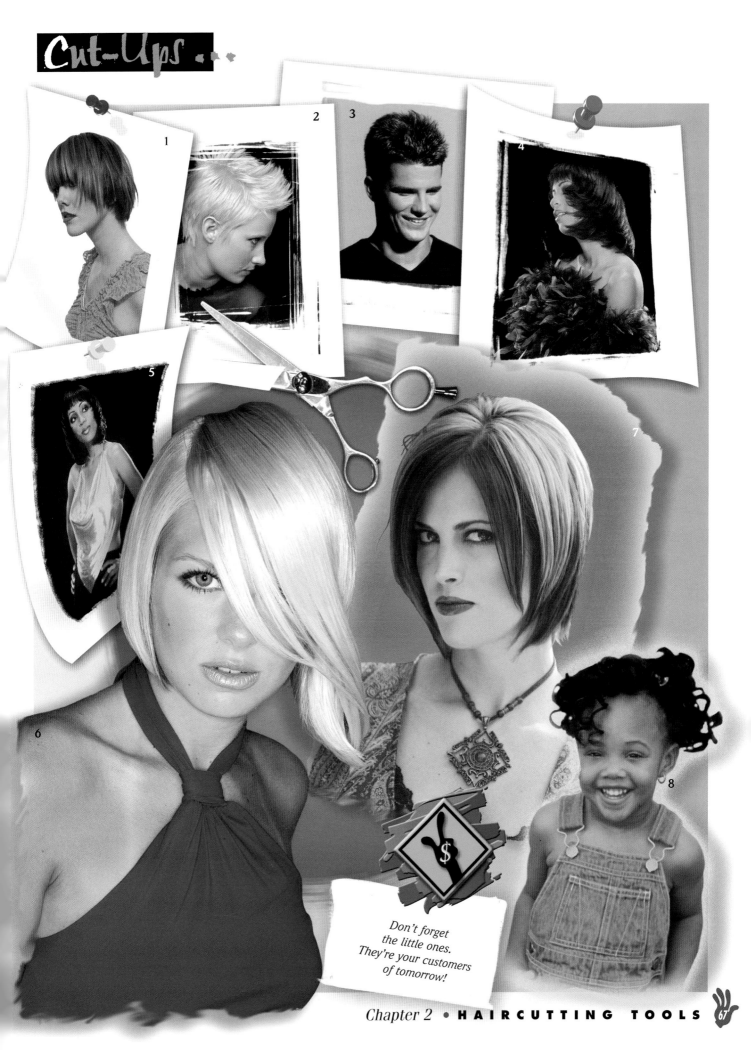

Cut-Ups...

1

2

3

4

5

6

7

8

Don't forget
the little ones.
They're your customers
of tomorrow!

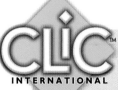

Haircutting Tools REVIEW QUESTIONS

TRUE OR FALSE

_F_   1. When airforming or cutting hair, the elbows should always be close to the body.

_F_   2. There should always be a space between the concentrator and the brush when airforming.

_T_   3. The more teeth per scissors, the less hair will be removed when cutting.

_T_   4. The screw head of the scissors should face toward you when cutting.

_F_   5. Hair should always be dry before razor cutting.

_F_   6. A water-based disinfectant is recommended for cleaning scissor blades.

_T_   7. The guard should be used to help insert and remove razor blades whenever possible, for safety.

_F_   8. Weave cut scissors are used to remove very small amounts of hair.

_T_   9. A thermal metal round brush retains the heat from the airformer to work in a manner similar to hot rollers or curling irons.

_T_   10. Cobalt scissors are not recommended, because they don't maintain a sharp cutting edge.

MULTIPLE CHOICE

1. Which clipper position is used to create elevations within a clipper cut?

    A. elevation position   **B.** upward arching position   C. angled position

2. Which scissors position is recommended for proper ergonomics and high-precision cutting?

    A. alternate   B. thumb down   **C.** thumb up

3. How often should scissors be lubricated?

    A. daily   B. monthly   C. hourly

4. Which comb is an excellent tool for men's flat top haircuts?

    A. shark tooth comb   B. rattail comb   **C.** clipper comb

5. Which airformer attachment is used to minimize airflow?

    A. diffuser   B. concentrator   C. minimizer

6. Which finger technique provides maximum pressure and hair removal when razor cutting?

    A. maximum finger technique   **B.** 3-finger technique   C. 1-finger technique

7. Which liquid styling tool is used to control curls, waves and damaged ends?

    A. smoothing lotion   B. pomade   C. finishing spray

8. When airforming, where should the airflow be directed?

    A. away from your body   **B.** toward the floor   C. into your body

9. Which blade of the scissors does the cutting?

    A. moving blade   **B.** still blade   C. alternate blade

10. When cutting scissors over comb, what is the relationship between the two tools?

    A. perpendicular   B. together   **C.** parallel

STUDENT'S NAME   DATE   GRADE

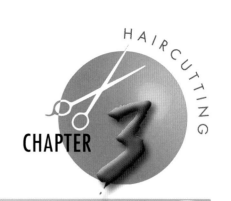

great masses
facial shapes
density patterns
proportions

counterbalance
anthropometry
anatomy

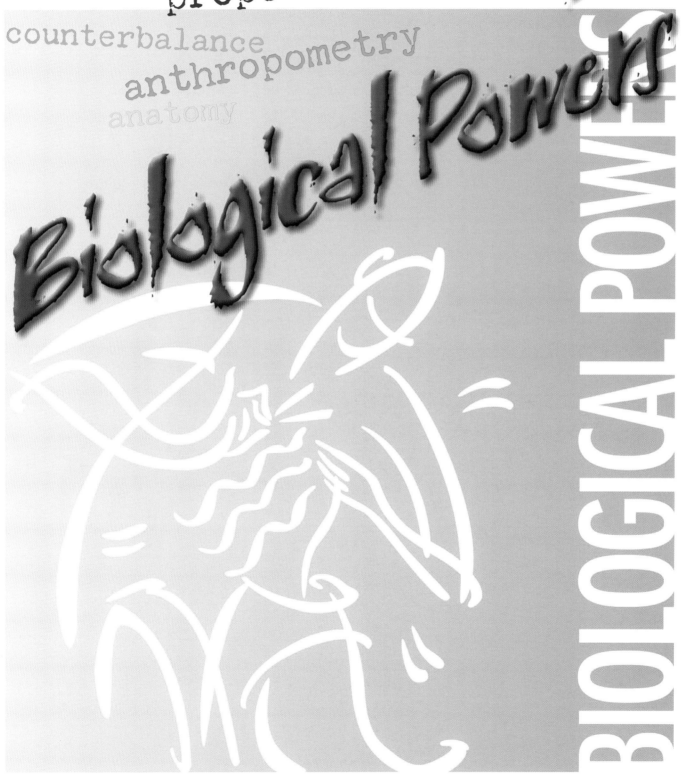

Biological Powers

BIOLOGICAL POWERS

All fine architectural designs begin with a concept. As a haircutting architect, you must develop a cutting concept prior to executing the haircut. Using information from your client consultation combined with your own creativity is very important in formulating your haircut concept. However, your concept must have an anthropometrical foundation.

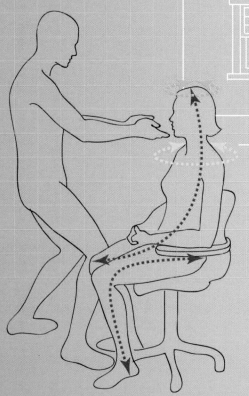

Anthropometry is the study of human body measurements for examination and comparison purposes. Specifically, the individual's height, weight and body shape must be considered when conceptualizing the perfect cut for each client. These are important factors which will either be accented or counterbalanced to provide a well-proportioned, harmonious end result.

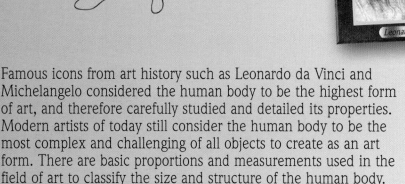

Leonardo Da Vinci

Michelangelo

Famous icons from art history such as Leonardo da Vinci and Michelangelo considered the human body to be the highest form of art, and therefore carefully studied and detailed its properties. Modern artists of today still consider the human body to be the most complex and challenging of all objects to create as an art form. There are basic proportions and measurements used in the field of art to classify the size and structure of the human body.

Your role as a professional haircutter is to evaluate the existing body shape and measurements to determine the most flattering, proportionate cut for each client. In this chapter we will examine the individual components of the human body and, specifically, the head in order to provide an overview of the elements of evaluation. Through practice and experimentation, you will develop your own method and intuition for this evaluation and recommendation process.

Proportions and Symmetry...

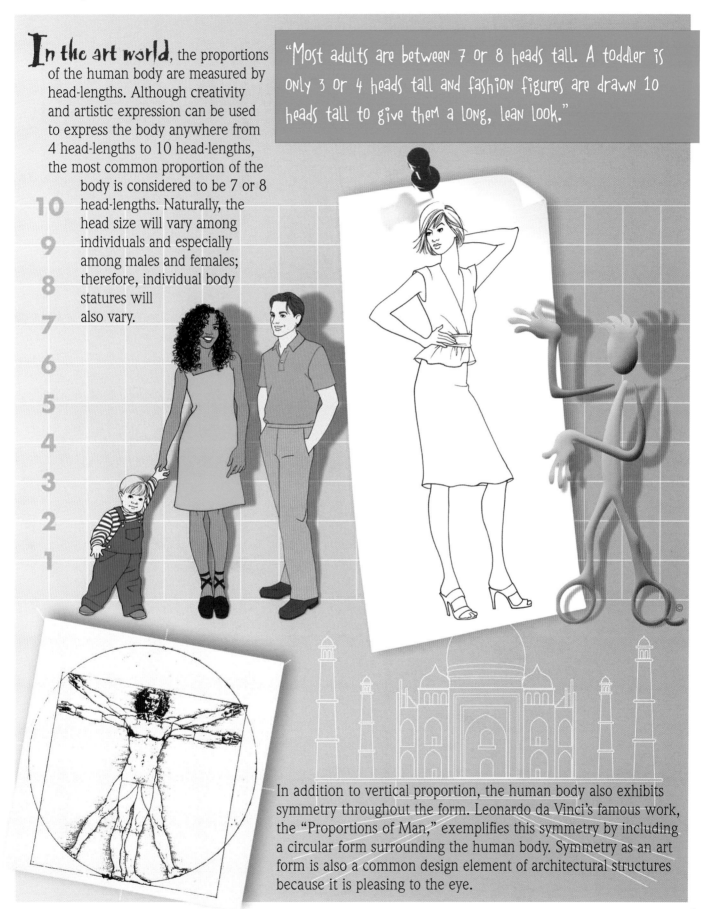

In the art world, the proportions of the human body are measured by head-lengths. Although creativity and artistic expression can be used to express the body anywhere from 4 head-lengths to 10 head-lengths, the most common proportion of the body is considered to be 7 or 8 head-lengths. Naturally, the head size will vary among individuals and especially among males and females; therefore, individual body statures will also vary.

"Most adults are between 7 or 8 heads tall. A toddler is only 3 or 4 heads tall and fashion figures are drawn 10 heads tall to give them a long, lean look."

In addition to vertical proportion, the human body also exhibits symmetry throughout the form. Leonardo da Vinci's famous work, the "Proportions of Man," exemplifies this symmetry by including a circular form surrounding the human body. Symmetry as an art form is also a common design element of architectural structures because it is pleasing to the eye.

Body Shape ...

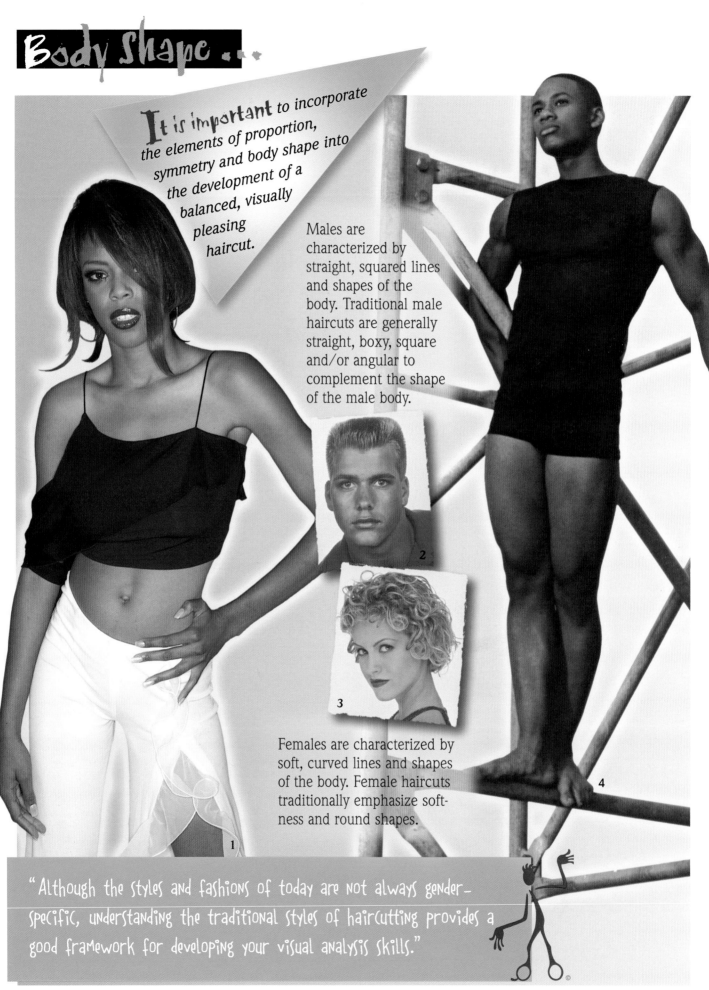

It is important to incorporate the elements of proportion, symmetry and body shape into the development of a balanced, visually pleasing haircut.

Males are characterized by straight, squared lines and shapes of the body. Traditional male haircuts are generally straight, boxy, square and/or angular to complement the shape of the male body.

2

3

Females are characterized by soft, curved lines and shapes of the body. Female haircuts traditionally emphasize softness and round shapes.

1

4

"Although the styles and fashions of today are not always gender-specific, understanding the traditional styles of haircutting provides a good framework for developing your visual analysis skills."

Body Shape ...

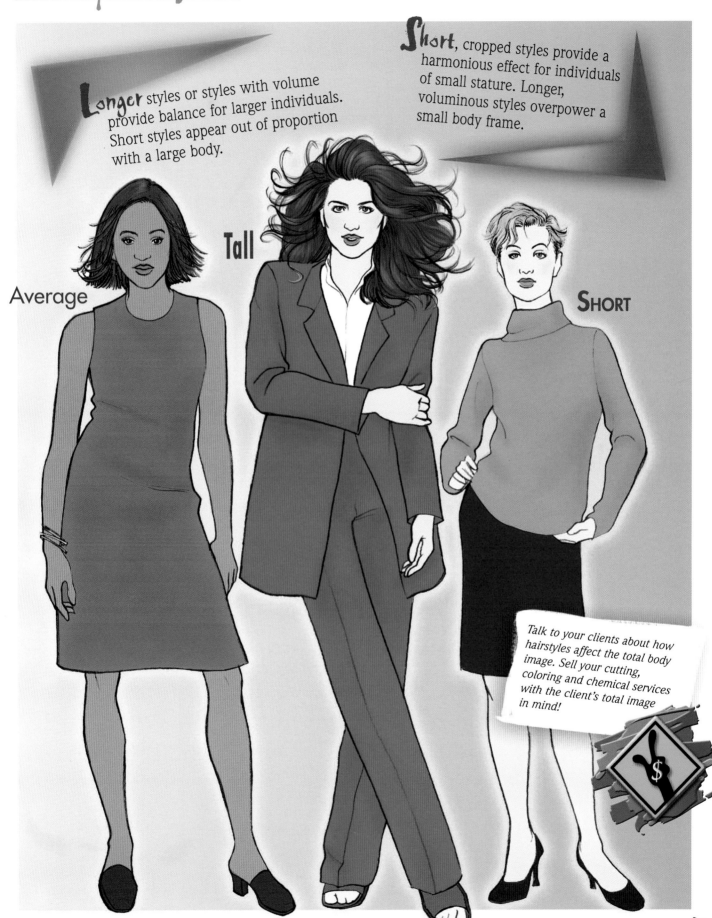

Longer styles or styles with volume provide balance for larger individuals. Short styles appear out of proportion with a large body.

Short, cropped styles provide a harmonious effect for individuals of small stature. Longer, voluminous styles overpower a small body frame.

Average

Tall

Short

Talk to your clients about how hairstyles affect the total body image. Sell your cutting, coloring and chemical services with the client's total image in mind!

Anatomy of the Head ...

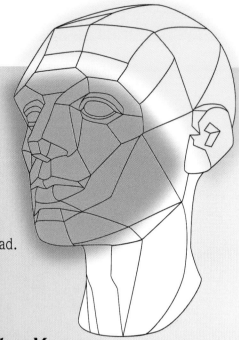

In addition to visualizing the entire body size, shape and proportions, a detailed examination of the head is a critical element to consider when formulating the most appropriate haircut for each client.

The head consists of two major masses, called <u>The Great Masses</u>.

▷ <u>THE CRANIAL MASS</u> – the ball shape of the top of the head.

▶ <u>THE FACE</u> – a tapered, cylindrical shape.

The facial area consists of the following nine <u>Secondary Masses</u>:

1 The brow

2 The tapered wedge of the nose

3 The cheek bone

4 The eye socket

5 The barrel of the mouth

6 The box of the chin

7 The angle of the lower jaw, or jaw point

8 The side arch of the cheek bone

9 The shell of the ear

The shape and placement of the secondary masses of the head must be contemplated during the initial client consultation and evaluation. The general appearance of the client's face and head are directly influenced by the secondary masses.

"When viewing a client's profile, the cranial mass ends at the bridge of the nose under the brow."

Zones of the Head ...

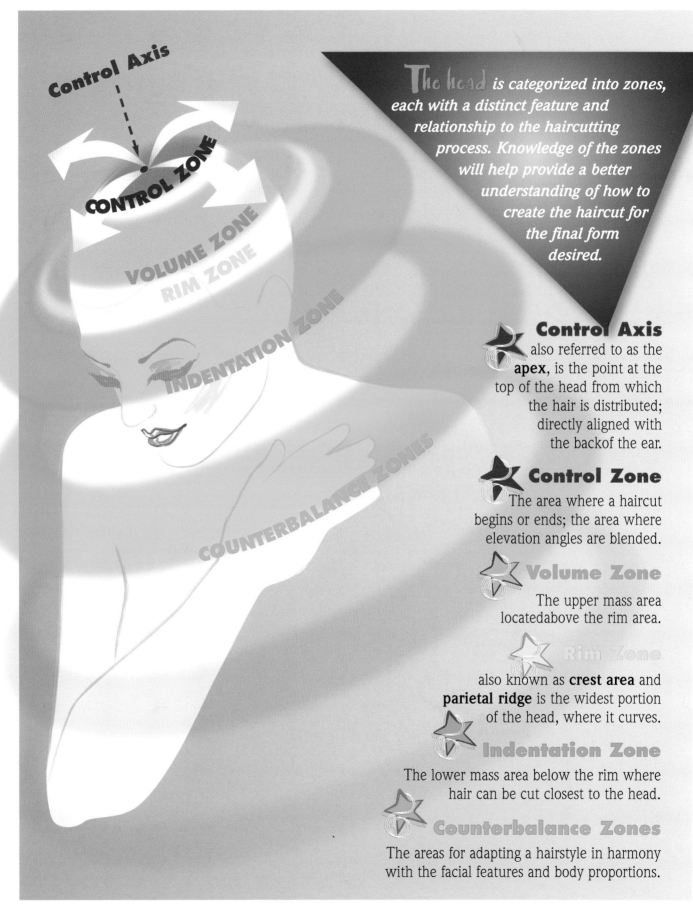

Control Axis

CONTROL ZONE

VOLUME ZONE

RIM ZONE

INDENTATION ZONE

COUNTERBALANCE ZONES

The head is categorized into zones, each with a distinct feature and relationship to the haircutting process. Knowledge of the zones will help provide a better understanding of how to create the haircut for the final form desired.

Control Axis
also referred to as the **apex**, is the point at the top of the head from which the hair is distributed; directly aligned with the backof the ear.

Control Zone
The area where a haircut begins or ends; the area where elevation angles are blended.

Volume Zone
The upper mass area locatedabove the rim area.

Rim Zone
also known as **crest area** and **parietal ridge** is the widest portion of the head, where it curves.

Indentation Zone
The lower mass area below the rim where hair can be cut closest to the head.

Counterbalance Zones
The areas for adapting a hairstyle in harmony with the facial features and body proportions.

Shapes of Hair...

Constructing the Haircut

Building Blocks

Cutting hair is like constructing a building. Both must be built with a strong foundation, quality materials, good workmanship and attention to details. If a building is not built properly, it will collapse, as if made of sand.

The structural building blocks of haircutting are the individual characteristics of each client's hair that you work with. In order to create each individual haircut, the following characteristics must be considered: the shape and texture of the hair, the density, the growth patterns and the health and condition of the hair.

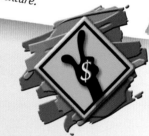

Use the characteristics of each client's hair to guide your retailing efforts. Suggest the retail products that will enhance the client's hair condition and texture.

Following is a checklist of the building blocks of constructing a haircut:

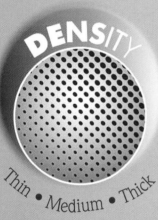

DENSITY

Thin • Medium • Thick

Examine:
- the hair density: thin, medium or thick
- the hair growth patterns and movement
- the hair shapes: straight, wavy or curly
- the hair condition: healthy, dry, oily, damaged or chemically treated

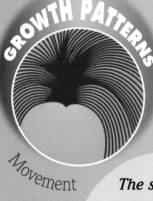

GROWTH PATTERNS

Movement

Shape

Straight • Wavy • Curly

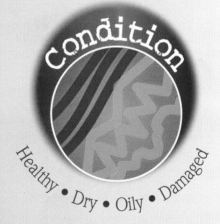

Condition

Healthy • Dry • Oily • Damaged

The shape and condition of the hair will guide you in the construction of a haircut that will work best for your client's lifestyle.

"Work with the natural hair shape, texture and growth pattern - not against it!"

76 HAIRCUTTING

Shapes of Hair...

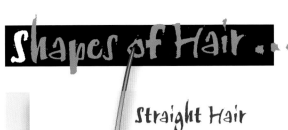

Straight Hair
Takes the form of a circle.

Wavy Hair
Takes the form of a large oval.

Curly Hair
Takes the form of a narrow oval.

Follicle Shape

Hair is broadly classified into three forms: straight, wavy and curly.

The form of each strand of hair is determined by the shape of its follicle.
Forms emerge as the hair exits the follicle at the scalp.

Each individual has a unique production and growth rate, size and shape of the hair. These factors are also influenced by ethnicity. The following are generalities about hair according to ethnic group:

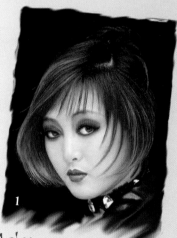

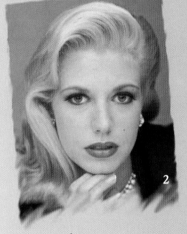

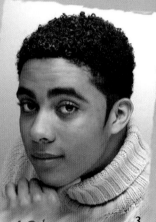

Asian
Asian hair is the thickest and most coarse hair of all ethnic groups. Cross-section examination almost always reveals circular follicle shapes. The density of follicles is less than Caucasians, ranging from 90,000 to 120,000.

Caucasian
Caucasian hair occurs in all three forms: straight, wavy and curly. Cross-section examination reveals circular or oval follicle shapes. The density of follicles on the scalp ranges from 100,000 to 150,000 per person and varies in relationship to natural hair color. Red-haired individuals have the least density of hair growth, followed by brunettes with average hair growth, and blondes have the greatest density.

African
African hair is often tightly-coiled or spiral hair. Cross-section examination reveals elliptical and sometimes even flat, ribbon-like follicle shapes. This provides great strength and rigidity to the hair across the widest area and pliability across the narrow area of the strand, creating the natural flexing and coiling motion of the hair. Scalp density is very similar to Caucasian hair.

Hair Growth Patterns

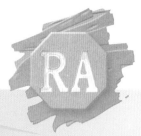

Examination of hair growth patterns is an important component of hair analysis. Areas such as cowlicks may need special consideration in order to achieve the desired style. Cutting with natural growth directions will help to minimize difficulties in styling. It is also important to carefully determine the amount of tension used for cutting strong growth pattern areas, to prevent the hair from becoming too short.

Hairlines

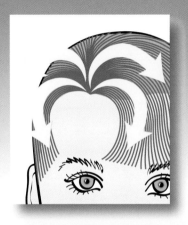

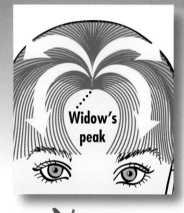

Widow's peak

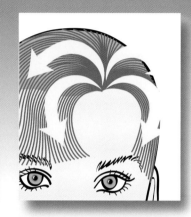

Napes

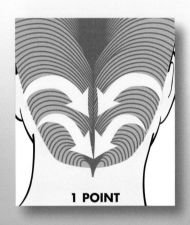

1 POINT

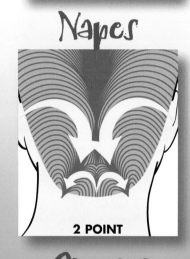

2 POINT

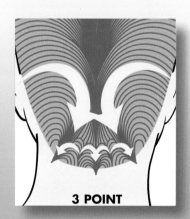

3 POINT

Crowns

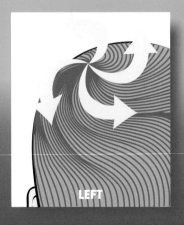

LEFT

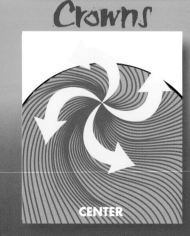

CENTER

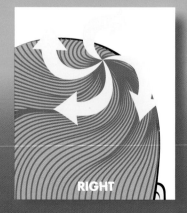

RIGHT

Hair Density Patterns

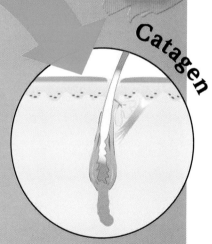

THICK · · · · · · · · THIN
THIN · · · · · · CROWN
HAIRLINE
THICK
NAPE
THIN

Individual strands of hair grow and are lost simultaneously and at varying rates on each person's head at all times. The resulting hair density of each individual will affect the ability to achieve volume in a hairstyle and should therefore be considered in the conceptualization and planning stages of the haircut. Density patterns are different in males than in females.

Anagen

Hair Growth

The hair growth cycle consists of three phases:

Hair is typically thinner in the crown, hairline and nape areas.

The period of active growth

This cycle

is repeated numerous times and in different sequences within the follicles on our heads. Therefore, at any one point in time, on average we have only 90% of the hair on our heads. The remaining 10% of the follicles are in the resting stage. As long as hair loss is balanced with new hair growth, overall density will not visibly change. Average daily hair loss is between 30 and 50 strands of hair per person. If hair loss exceeds 100 strands per day, new growth will not be able to adequately replace the losses and baldness occurs. Natural hair loss is also affected seasonally, with more hair being shed in the autumn and the spring than the summer. This is directly related to sunlight and weather conditions.

Catagen

The period of breakdown and change

Telogen

The resting period before growth resumes

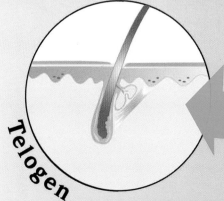

"Did you know that hair grows fastest during the teens and early 20's? Also, hair growth slows as the length increases. Pretty interesting!"

Hair Loss...

Hair loss can be caused by any one or a combination of the following factors:

- Heredity
- Toxic substances
- Severe radiation
- Nervous disorder
- Hormonal imbalance
- Illness and infectious disease
- Aging
- Injury and impairment

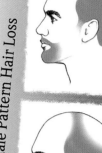
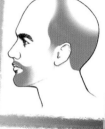
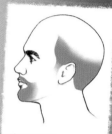
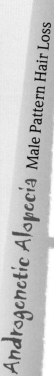

Androgenetic Alopecia Male Pattern Hair Loss

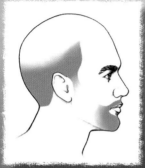
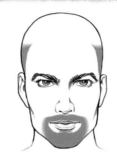
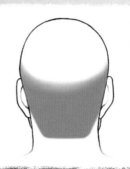

Male Hair Loss

Typical male pattern baldness is also known as Hippocratic Baldness, named in honor of Hippocrates and his own baldness pattern and lifelong search for the cure. It normally starts before age 40 and first occurs along the frontal hairline and in the crown area

In order to inherit baldness, a male needs only one gene – either one from the mother's side of the family or one from the father's side.

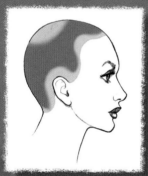
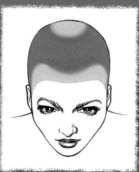
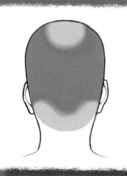

Female Hair Loss

Baldness in women usually occurs more evenly throughout the upper 2/3 of the head.

A female needs to inherit two genes – one from the mother's side of the family and one from the father's side – in order to develop baldness.

"Since males only have to inherit one gene for baldness, we see more bald males than females."

According to the International Society of Hair Restoration Surgery (www.ishrs.org), an estimated 35 million men in the United States are affected by male pattern hair loss. The male hormone, testosterone, causes hair loss in men who carry the gene for hair loss. Testosterone is converted to DHT, which enters the hair follicles and alters the production of proteins. This ultimately causes hair growth to stop completely. Hair loss is first noticeable in the recession areas, and later in the crown area. As the hair loss progresses, the two areas are eventually joined into one large area, as shown above.

Hair Loss Products ...

Advancements in medical and scientific technology have provided some exciting treatments for people who experience hair loss. Two of the current most popular treatments are Rogaine® and Propecia®. However, scientific research is ongoing in the area, and new treatment alternatives are sure to emerge in the future.

The customer's needs always come first. Make referrals to other professionals for areas beyond your training and knowledge. This added service and caring will help strengthen your customer's loyalty!

Rogaine®

The active ingredient in Rogaine®, Minoxidil, was approved by the FDA in 1988 as a safe and effective treatment for male and female hair loss and thinning. Originally used to treat high blood pressure, Minoxidil was discovered to also stimulate hair growth and thickness by invigorating shrunken hair follicles and increasing their size.

Rogaine® is a topical liquid solution that is applied twice daily prior to the use of any styling products. Special care should be taken in conjunction with the use of Rogaine® to prevent scalp irritation. Mild shampoo should be used for cleansing, and the use of Rogaine® is not recommended prior to receiving chemical services in the salon.

Visit www.rogaine.com for additional information

Propecia®

Unlike Rogaine®, Propecia® is taken once daily in pill form. Finasteride, the active ingredient, blocks the formation of DHT, the hormone causing male pattern baldness. This blockage occurs by disabling the enzyme that is present in and around the hair follicles of balding men.

Propecia® does not seem to grow hair in areas that are completely bald. Therefore, its main benefit is the ability to reduce or terminate hair loss, or regrow hair in parts of the scalp with thin density.

Visit www.propecia.com for additional information.

Shapes of the Face . . .

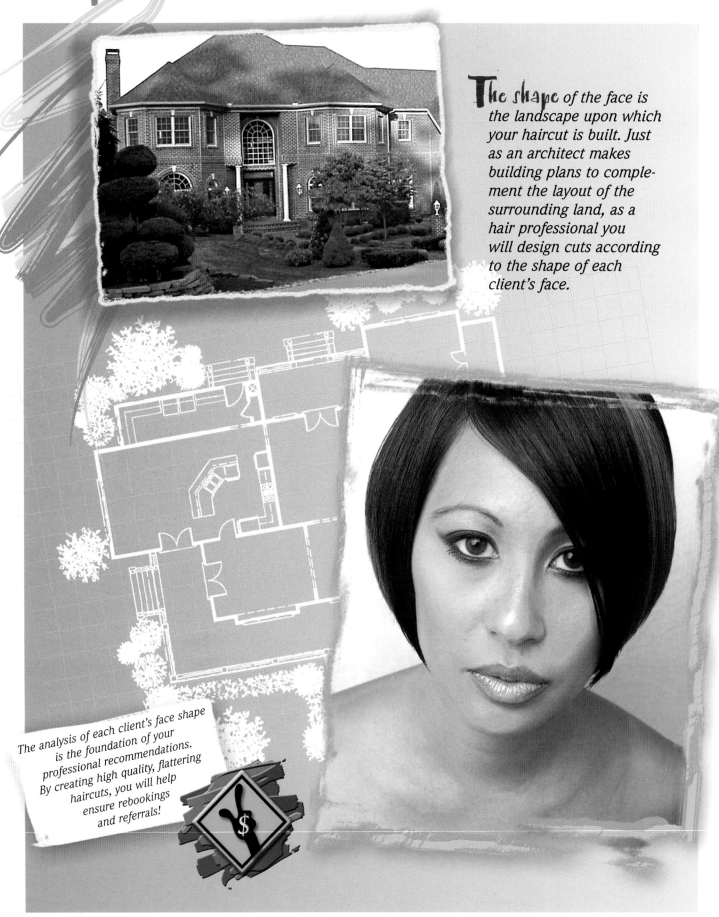

The shape of the face is the landscape upon which your haircut is built. Just as an architect makes building plans to complement the layout of the surrounding land, as a hair professional you will design cuts according to the shape of each client's face.

The analysis of each client's face shape is the foundation of your professional recommendations. By creating high quality, flattering haircuts, you will help ensure rebookings and referrals!

The Classic Oval . . .

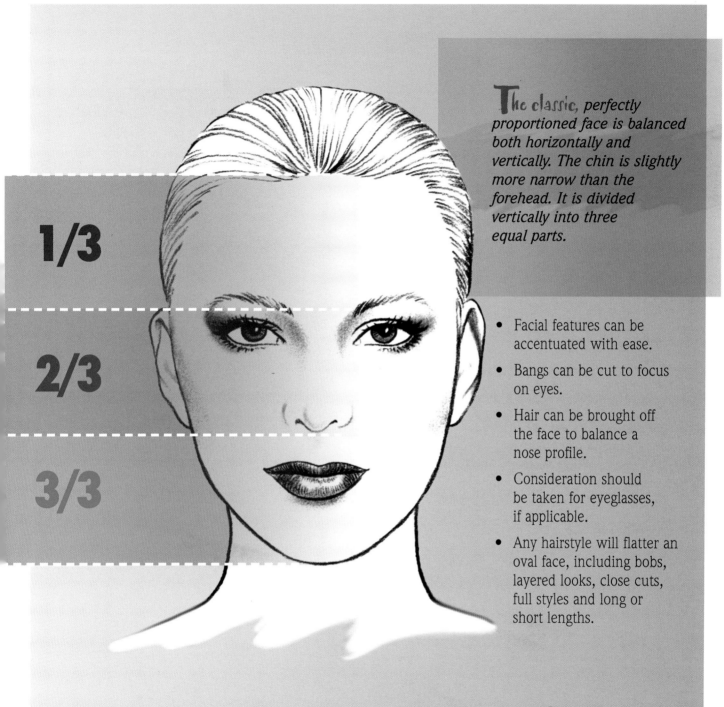

1/3

2/3

3/3

The classic, *perfectly proportioned face is balanced both horizontally and vertically. The chin is slightly more narrow than the forehead. It is divided vertically into three equal parts.*

- Facial features can be accentuated with ease.
- Bangs can be cut to focus on eyes.
- Hair can be brought off the face to balance a nose profile.
- Consideration should be taken for eyeglasses, if applicable.
- Any hairstyle will flatter an oval face, including bobs, layered looks, close cuts, full styles and long or short lengths.

"Do you want to check out your own face shape and facial proportions? Stand very close to a mirror, pull all your hair straight back tightly, then trace the outline and divisions of your face with removable marker or old lipstick. Step back and study the marks on the mirror. What face shape do you have?"

Shapes of the Face ...

RA

The following guidelines *will help you create balanced, visually pleasing hairstyles. Keep in mind that to correct and enhance any of the facial shapes, the primary objective is to use the hairstyle to create the illusion of an oval-shaped face.*

Round

The round face is wide with a rounded jaw line and hairline. Hairstyles should create an illusion of length in the face.

- Use minimal volume at the sides.
- Add height to the crown.

Oblong

The oblong face is long and narrow. Hairstyles should shorten and widen the appearance of the face.

- Add volume to the sides, for width.
- Bangs can be used to help shorten the facial appearance.
- Keep the overall length short to moderate.

Square

The forehead and jaw line of the square face are almost equal in width. Hairstyles should add softness to the facial contour.
- Use volume on the sides.
- Soften the facial frame by styling the hair toward the face.
- Asymmetrical styles can be used if the facial features are well-balanced.

Diamond

The diamond face has a high, narrow forehead, wide cheekbones and a pointed chin. Hairstyles should reduce the width of the cheeks and soften the vertical length of the face.

- Add fullness to the forehead and chin areas.
- Keep hair close to the head at the sides.
- Do not lift the hair away from the sides at the cheekbone areas.

Triangle / Pear

The triangle/pear face has a narrow forehead and a wide jaw line. Hairstyles should expand the width of the forehead and disguise the jaw area.
- Add width with volume in the forehead and crown areas.
- Use a soft bang to disguise the forehead.
- Style the hair toward the chin and jaw areas .

Inverted Triangle / Heart

The inverted triangle/heart face has a wide forehead with a narrow jaw and chin area. Hairstyles should add volume to the jaw line and conceal the width of the forehead.
- Use a soft, partial fringe to offset the width of the forehead.
- Minimize volume in the forehead and crown areas.
- Use volume in the jaw and chin areas.

Shapes of the Face ...

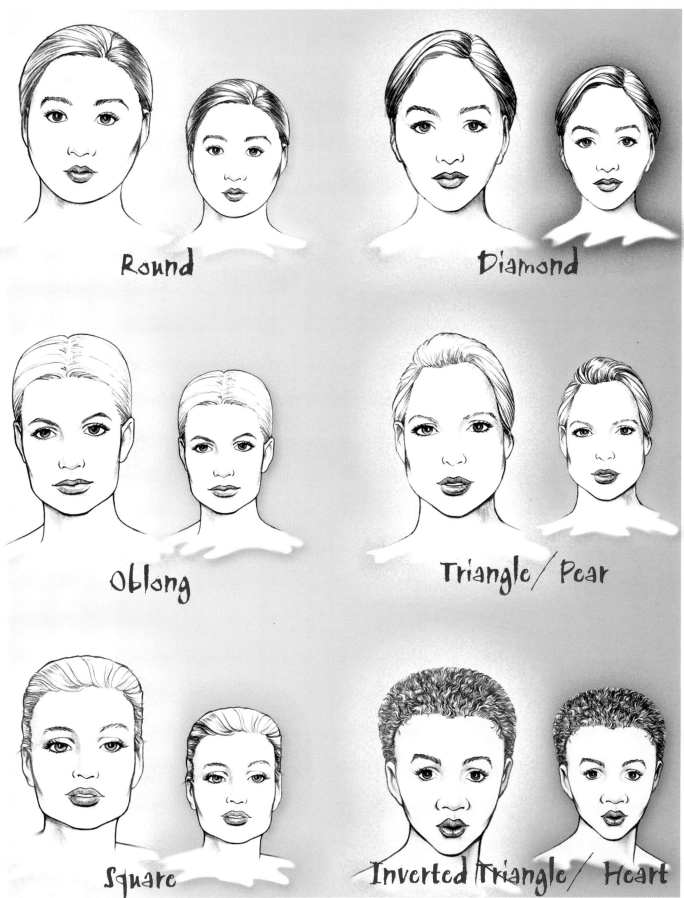

Round

Diamond

Oblong

Triangle / Pear

Square

Inverted Triangle / Heart

Counterbalances . . .

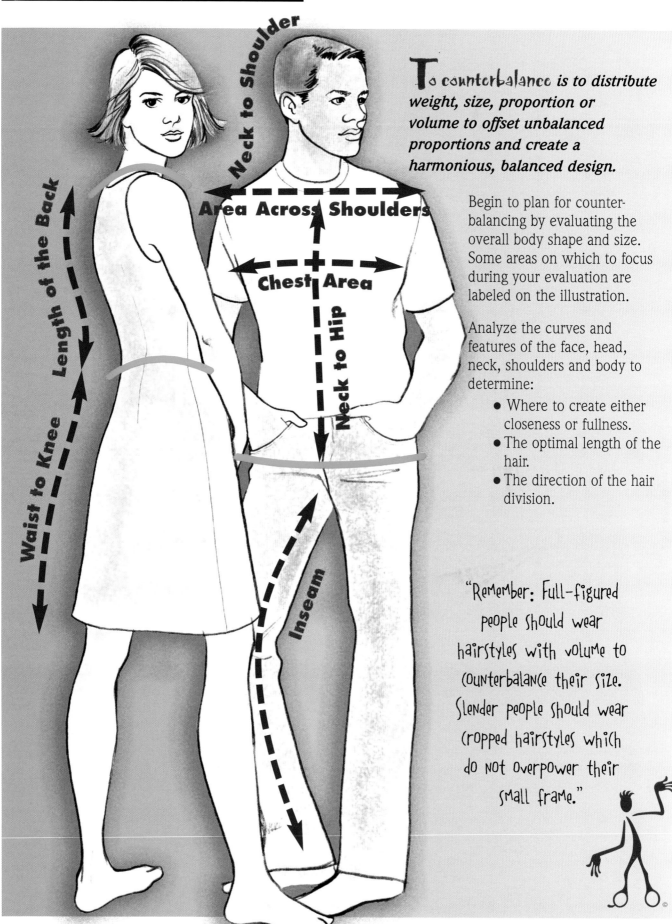

Neck to Shoulder

Area Across Shoulders

Chest Area

Neck to Hip

Length of the Back

Waist to Knee

Inseam

To counterbalance *is to distribute weight, size, proportion or volume to offset unbalanced proportions and create a harmonious, balanced design.*

Begin to plan for counter-balancing by evaluating the overall body shape and size. Some areas on which to focus during your evaluation are labeled on the illustration.

Analyze the curves and features of the face, head, neck, shoulders and body to determine:

- Where to create either closeness or fullness.
- The optimal length of the hair.
- The direction of the hair division.

"Remember: Full-figured people should wear hairstyles with volume to counterbalance their size. Slender people should wear cropped hairstyles which do not overpower their small frame."

Counterbalances . . .

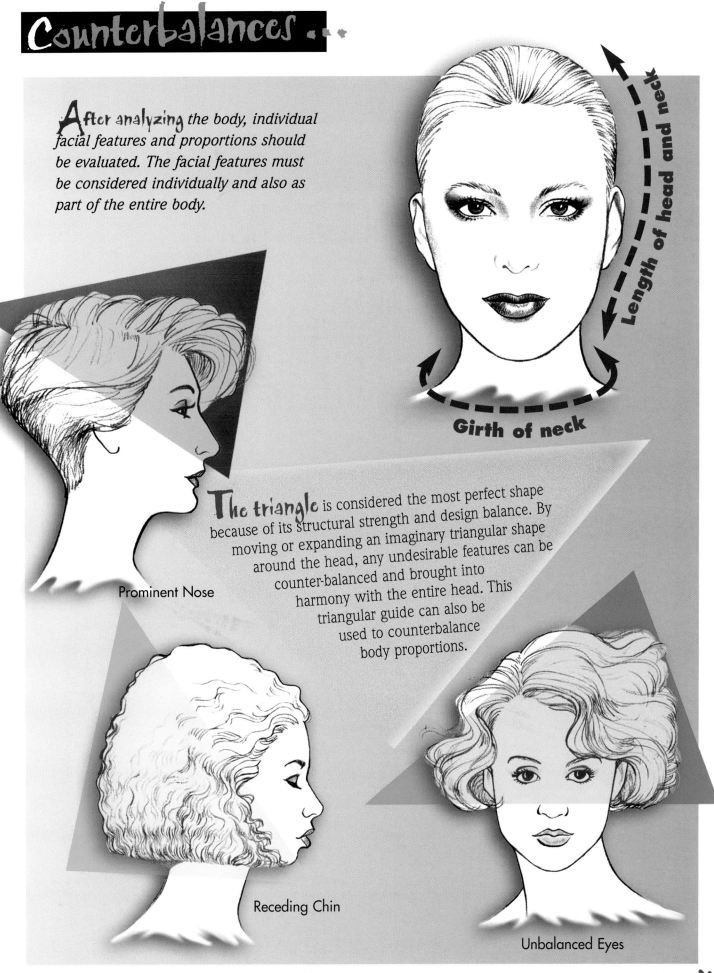

After analyzing the body, individual facial features and proportions should be evaluated. The facial features must be considered individually and also as part of the entire body.

Length of head and neck

Girth of neck

Prominent Nose

The triangle is considered the most perfect shape because of its structural strength and design balance. By moving or expanding an imaginary triangular shape around the head, any undesirable features can be counter-balanced and brought into harmony with the entire head. This triangular guide can also be used to counterbalance body proportions.

Receding Chin

Unbalanced Eyes

Counterbalancing . . .

the top third
of the face

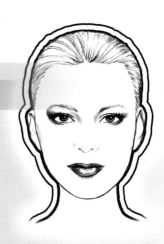

Following are guidelines for counterbalancing facial features in the top third of the face – the FOREHEAD and EYE area.

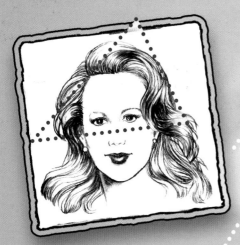

Close Set Eyes

Use an off-center triangle and place the base below the eyes and the upper tip on one of the sides of the face. Move the triangle position up or down depending upon the individual's face shape. The triangle should be in a lower position for long, rectangular faces and in an upper position for oval- and round-shaped faces. Design the hair with fullness and open up the face at the temple area.

Wide Set Eyes

Place the base of a balanced triangle across the eyes with the upper tip at the top of the frontal area. This creates upward distance from the eyes, adding length to a round face. Reverse the position of the triangle for individuals with a square-shaped face. Design the hair with a partial, lifted bang.

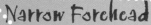

Narrow Forehead

Place the tip of a balanced triangle at the bridge of the nose or the front of the hairline (depending upon the shortness of the forehead) and the base framing the outer perimeter of the crown area. Cut the hair short to mid-length with design elements moving away from the face. Add fullness in the volume area to offset the small size of the forehead.

Wide Forehead

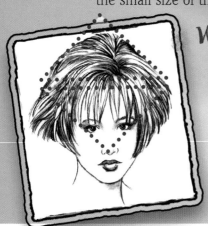

Place the base of a balanced triangle across the front hairline and the tip at the top of the crown area for round-faced individuals. Put the tip of the triangle at the bridge of the nose for long, rectangular-shaped faces. Use two triangles base-to-base (a diamond shape) as the balance guide for all other face shapes. Always place a soft fringe (bangs) onto the side areas of the forehead to conceal some of the width.

Following are guidelines *for counterbalancing facial features in the center third of the face—the NOSE area.*

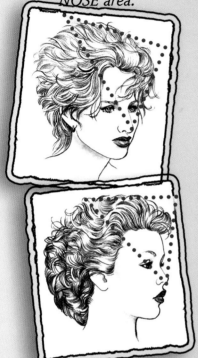

Large Nose

Place an off-center triangle with the base running from the tip of the nose to the top of the frontal bang area and the tip of the triangle at the back crown area. Place volume in the front forehead and the high occipital and crown areas. Create softness around the frontal fringe area.

Small Nose

Place a balanced triangle in the front third of the head, with the tips at the tip of the nose, the frontal area and the control axis. Design hair with movement in the frontal third drawn off the face. This gives the illusion of action within the hairdesign, and detracts from a child-like nose.

Wide and/or Flat Nose

Place two balanced triangles back-to-back in a diamond shape with the bases at the outer perimeter of the head and the tips at the nose and crown areas. Design the hair close on the sides, and moving away from the face. Work in symmetrical shapes to elongate or slenderize the shape of the nose.

Bent or Crooked Nose

Place an asymmetrical triangle with the tip in the frontal area of the head directly above the arch of the eyebrow and the base along the collar area, or lower for square or rectangular faces. Design the movement of the hair to flow asymmetrically across the face to draw attention away from the nose. Avoid using a center part, which draws the eye to the center division of the face (and therefore the nose).

Long Nose

Place the tip of a balanced triangle at the control axis and the base at the bottom of the chin or collar area. Design the hair with volume and width to create a full shape close, short cuts will only accentuate long and narrow features. Avoid even design components and center partings.

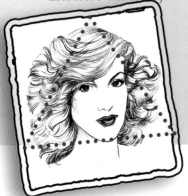

Counterbalancing... the bottom third of the face

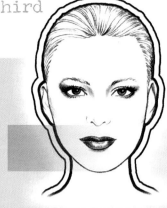

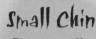 Following are guidelines *for counterbalancing facial features in the bottom third of the face–the JAW and CHIN area.*

Small Chin

Place an off-center triangle with points at the chin, frontal area and crown area. Cut hair to collar-length in the nape area and raise the crown area to add softness and depth from a profile view.

Large Chin

Place an off-center triangle with points at the chin, back crown area and the bottom of the nape area. Length and volume in the nape area provide counterbalance to a large chin. However, depending upon the shape of the chin (square, round or triangular), a smaller triangle with a shorter hair length in the nape will also work.

Square Jaw

Place a balanced triangle in an off-center position with the tip in the control area and the base in the jaw area. Design the hair to frame the face in curved elements to add softness to the face.

Round Jaw

Place a balanced triangle in an off-center position with the tip aligned with the arch of the eyebrow and the base along the jaw area. Design the hair in an asymmetric style using straight lines to distract from the curvature of the chin area.

Long Jaw

Place a tall, balanced triangle with the tip at the control point and the base along the collar bone area. Hair should be long and designed with fullness to counterbalance the length of the jaw line.

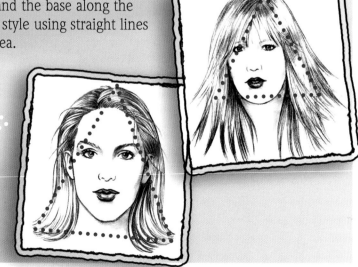

Counterbalancing

A profile is the outline, shape or silhouette of the side view of the face. There are three standard profiles: STRAIGHT, CONCAVE and CONVEX. The following counterbalance guidelines will assist in creating flattering, appropriate hairstyles for your clients.

Straight

The ideal profile is straight, which is characterized by only slight curves of the face. Generally, all hairstyles are flattering to those with straight profiles and balanced facial features. The imaginary design triangle can begin at any point from the tip of the nose to the end of the chin and be used as a guideline for a balanced style.

Concave

A concave profile has a prominent forehead and strong chin, with the other facial features appearing to recede in comparison. An asymmetrical design triangle should be used to counterbalance concave features. The points of the triangle create the following effects:

- Move hair softly off the forehead.
- Direct hair away from the chin area.
- Create a soft, upward design in the back crown area.
- Create volume in the nape area to balance the protruding chin.

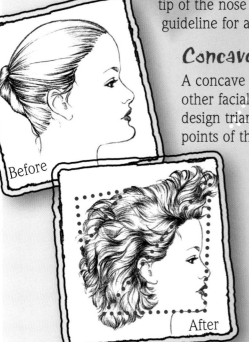

Before

After

Convex

A convex profile has a high hairline and receding chin area, creating an outwardly-rounded profile. The points of the design triangle are areas of special attention, as follows:

- Add volume and lift to the bangs.
- Keep cuts short to mid-length.
- Draw hair toward the face and chin area.
- Add volume to the crown area if it is flat.(optional)

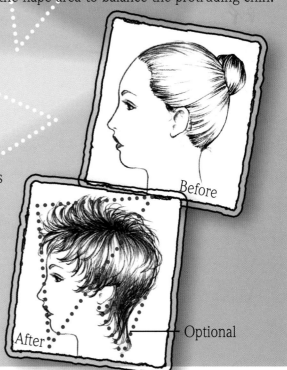

Before

After

Optional

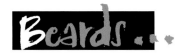

Beards...

The male beard has been a statement of fashion throughout history. It can help re-design the shape of the face and also camouflage imperfections. Understanding the basic points of how to grow and care for a beard will help you advise clients who already have, or are considering wearing a beard.

Growing a Beard

As a haircare professional, your male clients may consult you for advice about growing a beard. Or, you may recommend a beard to certain clients to enhance their look. The following advice will guide the beard growth process.

1 **Choose a good time.**
The best time to start a beard is during a vacation or extended weekend, when the client is less self-conscious about his appearance.

2 **Allow 4 to 6 weeks.**
Advise the client to stop shaving for the first 4 to 6 weeks. Letting the beard grow naturally will prevent over-trimming and over-shaping.

3 **Prevent itching.**
Itching may occur during the first several weeks. To minimize skin irritation, advise client to wash and condition the beard as it grows.

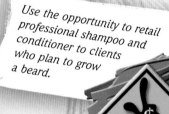

Use the opportunity to retail professional shampoo and conditioner to clients who plan to grow a beard.

Maintaining a Beard

Once the beard has grown to the desired length and density, a routine maintenance program must be established. You will play an important role in providing care at the salon as well as recommendations for at-home maintenance.

1 **Professional Shaping.**
The first shaping should be done at the salon. Likewise, re-shaping is recommended at all haircut appointments. Follow these guidelines:
  • Plot the boundaries with an eyebrow pencil.
  • Keeping the skin taut, use short strokes to shape the beard.
  • Carefully trim away from the penciled boundary or use an outline trimmer.
    Do NOT trim deeper than the boundary.
  • Use a trimmer to clean hair above the boundary.

2 **Maintenance Shaping.**
An electric or battery powered trimmer is a versatile tool for at-home trimming, shaping and shortening. The various guard attachments allow easy and precise shaping.

Consider stocking electric/battery powered trimmers in your retail area.

3 **Cleansing.**
Advise clients to clean their beards regularly with shampoo. It is recommended to shampoo the hair and beard at the same time.

4 **Conditioning.**
Recommend the use of a non-greasy conditioner to add softness and shine to the beard.

5 **Coloring.**
Offer haircolor to clients with gray in their beards, or with facial hair that is a different color from the hair on their head.

Counterbalancing with Beards...

Face size, shape and areas to be counterbalanced should be considered when helping a client choose a style of beard. Evaluate how different looks will accentuate the face and enhance the client's overall appearance. The following tips recommend beards to flatter particular face shapes and help hide imperfections.

Oval Face

Almost any beard or mustache is flattering to an oval face. Choose a style that will accentuate individual features. Longer, fuller beards tend to enhance larger features, while smaller features are accentuated by shorter beards.

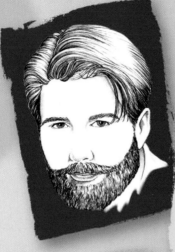

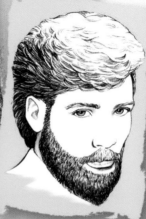

Round Face

Enhance a round face with a narrow beard. The vertical planes of the design draw the eye along the length of the face, rather than the width. A short, squared beard or triangular goatee also directs the eye to the vertical line of the face. Avoid short sideburns and thick beards, which emphasize the round shape of the face.

Square Face

Create a softer frame for a square face by choosing a rounded beard and mustache. Avoid sideburns, which frame the face and draw attention to the square shape.

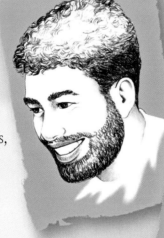

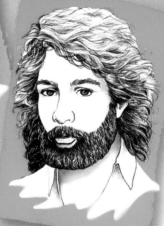

Oblong Face

Counterbalance an oblong (narrow) face with a beard that is fuller at the sides and shorter at the chin. Oblong faces are flattered by beards that create the illusion of an oval shape.

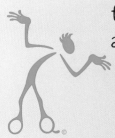

"Some additional points to consider when helping a client choose a beard:"

- A goatee can hide a pointy chin.
- A full beard can hide a double chin.
- A mustache can hide thin lips and soften a long or wide nose.
- A beard and/or mustache can help balance a balding hairline and draw attention away from the scalp.

Chapter 3 • **BIOLOGICAL POWERS** 93

Cutting Coordination and Control...

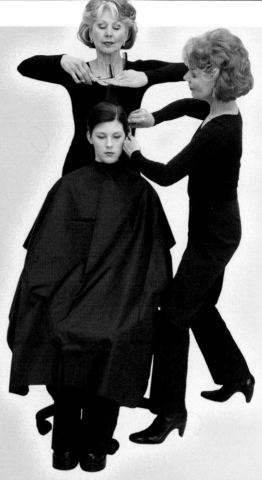

After evaluating the proportions and features of your client and formulating the appropriate cut, it is time to execute the cut. Now is the time to consider your own body! Personal comfort and control are influential to your cutting results. In order to develop precision haircutting skills, learning the coordination and control of the body, hands, scissors and feet positions is critical. It is through awareness and self-discipline that the necessary coordination is learned and becomes a professional working habit.

Body Position

Maintaining a disciplined yet relaxed body position will prevent fatigue while working. Imagine the center force of your body in the hip/pelvic area and "plant" yourself firmly in proper relationship to the client. Keep a slight bend in the knees to encourage good circulation and adjust your styling chair height as necessary to maintain an eye level view of the cutting process at all times while keeping your upper body straight from the waist up. Maintain flexibility and mobility by always keeping your elbows out and away from the body.

Position of Hands

The position of the hands in relationship to the client's head is an important element of precision haircutting. When holding the hair, the palm of the hand can either face outward, away from the head, or inward, toward the head. The position of the palm of the hand holding the hair being cut determines whether the cutting position is palm-to-palm or palm-to-scalp.

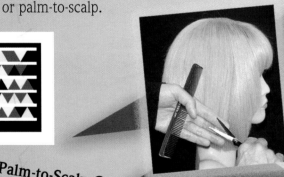

Palm-to-Palm Cutting Technique:

The palm faces outward. Using the palm-to-palm position when cutting prevents the hair from being lifted up off your hand and the hair from being pushed out of the front of the scissors. It also helps to direct the ends of the hair in the direction of the cutting line.

Palm-to-Scalp Cutting Technique:

The palm faces inward. Hand coordination and control is achieved when cutting higher degree cuts by using the palm to scalp hand position. Palm-to-scalp vertical cutting also helps turn the ends of the hair under.

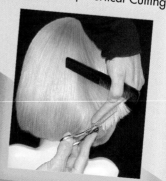

Palm-to-Scalp Vertical Cutting

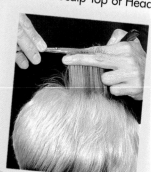

Palm-to-Scalp Top of Head

Maintain flexibility *in the wrists at all times to keep control of the hair and minimize trauma to the wrist area from overuse. Cumulative Trauma Disorders (CTDs) such as carpal tunnel syndrome and tendonitis can occur from the repetitive motions and overuse of the hands and wrists, especially in unnatural positions. An example is the twisting of the hand and wrist that occurs when cutting using the alternate position. This can not only contribute to the development of CTDs, but it will also affect the precision and quality of your cut.*

Alternate Position

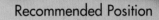

Recommended Position

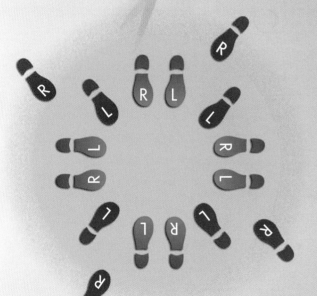

Position of Scissors

The position of the scissors is a natural extension of the position of your hands when cutting. This topic is discussed in greater detail in Chapter 2 on page 64.

Position of Feet

The stance of the haircutter is determined by the position of the feet during the cutting process. The feet should be parallel to each other and spaced shoulder-width apart to provide a solid, well-balanced foundation as you work. This is called **getting planted**. In addition, the feet should always be at a 90 degree angle to the edges of hair being cut. The illustrations of the basic feet positions will assist you in developing a practical, professional haircutting stance.

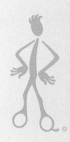

"In order to maintain proper body position and cutting control, your clothing must complement the tasks you perform. For example, clothing should not be too tight, too loose or baggy, skirts should not be too short, and tops should not be cropped or low cut. Use good judgment in selecting professional-looking attire that is flexibile and moves with you as you work."

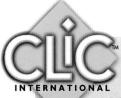

Biological Powers REVIEW QUESTIONS

MULTIPLE CHOICE

1. What is the name of the resting period in the hair growth cycle?
   A. telogen   B. resting   C. anagen

2. Which is the widest zone of the head, where it curves?
   A. major zone   B. rim zone   C. counterbalance zone

3. On average, how many strands of hair are lost per day?
   A. 6 to 10   B. 60 to 100   C. 30 to 50

4. What is the term for shifting weights and lengths of hair to create a well-proportioned style for the client?
   A. counterbalancing   B. proportioning   C. shifting

5. How many genes must a male inherit to develop baldness?
   A. 3   B. 2   C. 1

6. Which ethnic group generally has the thickest, most coarse hair?
   A. Asians   B. Caucasians   C. Europeans

7. What is the name of the ball shape on top of the head?
   A. secondary mass   B. cranial mass   C. ball mass

8. What is the term for studying human body measurements for examination and comparison purposes?
   A. examination   B. comparison   C. anthropometry

9. What shape is used as a guide to help counterbalance facial features?
   A. triangle   B. square   C. circle

10. What is the name of the prescription drug used to treat male pattern baldness?
    A. Propecia®   B. Rogaine®   C. Minoxidil

TRUE OR FALSE

F 1. Cutting against natural growth patterns will make styling the hair easier.

F 2. Hair density is usually thick in the hairline, crown and nape.

T 3. Beards can be used to hide or counterbalance male facial features.

T 4. The best position for comfort and precision haircutting is called getting planted.

T 5. The palm faces outward when cutting palm to palm.

F 6. There is nothing that can be done to prevent carpal tunnel syndrome. All haircutters will get it.

T 7. Male clients with beards present a good opportunity for maintenance visits for trimming or coloring services.

F 8. It isn't important to consider the profile of the face when counterbalancing. Only the head-on view needs to be counterbalanced.

F 9. A heart-shaped face is considered classic and perfectly proportioned. ~Oval

F 10. The face can be divided into four equal areas for examination and counterbalancing.

STUDENT'S NAME   DATE   GRADE

HAIRCUTTING 96

degrees

horizontal

elevation

diagonal

vertical

lines

progression

Mathematics of Haircutting

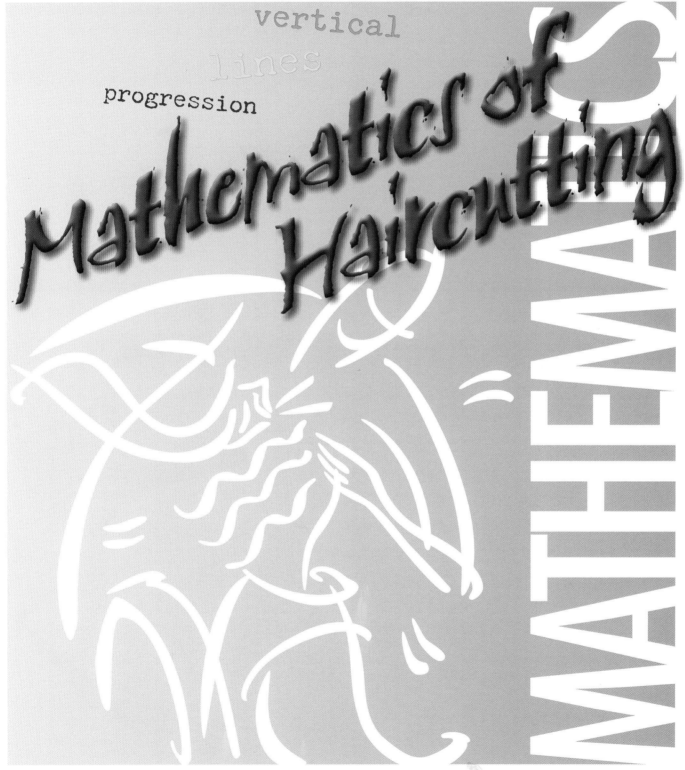

Architectural Haircutting...

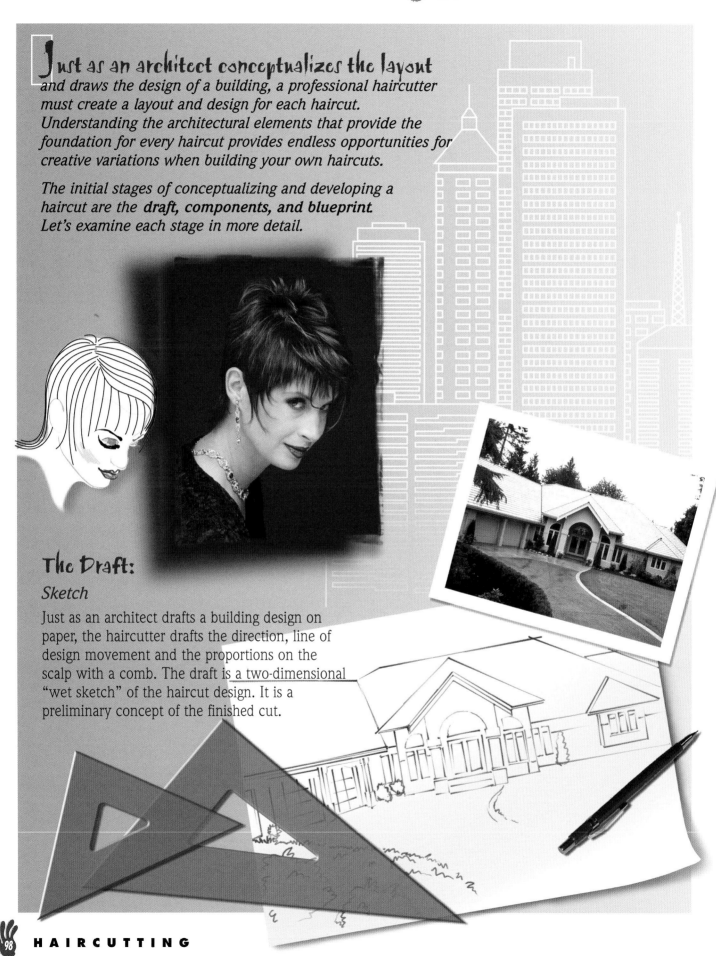

J ust as an architect conceptualizes the layout and draws the design of a building, a professional haircutter must create a layout and design for each haircut. Understanding the architectural elements that provide the foundation for every haircut provides endless opportunities for creative variations when building your own haircuts.

The initial stages of conceptualizing and developing a haircut are the **draft, components, and blueprint**. Let's examine each stage in more detail.

The Draft:

Sketch

Just as an architect drafts a building design on paper, the haircutter drafts the direction, line of design movement and the proportions on the scalp with a comb. The draft is a two-dimensional "wet sketch" of the haircut design. It is a preliminary concept of the finished cut.

Architectural Haircutting ...

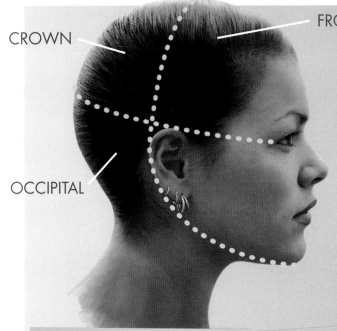

CROWN

FRONTAL

OCCIPITAL

The Components:

Areas

Walls, floors, ceilings, electrical wiring and plumbing are all basic components of every building. Likewise, there are basic components of every haircut. The head is divided into three main components for haircutting: the frontal area, the crown area and the occipital area. These areas are further divided into sections, subsections and partings according to the characteristics of each haircut.

The **frontal area** is the front area of the head from the highest point on the head to directly behind the ears, following the jawline.

The **crown area** is the upper back area of the head from below the highest point on the head to the top of the ears.

The **occipital area** is the lower back area of the head from below the top of the ears to the nape.

"An architect creates a blueprint of each building drawn to scale. For the haircutter, sectioning the head creates a similar blueprint of the individual components of the haircut."

The Blueprint:

Sections, sub-sections and partings

An architectural blueprint shows the room divisions and the details within each room of the building. For the haircutting professional, subsections and partings are the details within each section that customize a haircut.

Sections are defined areas that can be managed and controlled. **Sub-sections** are smaller divisions defined within a main section. **Partings** are even smaller linear divisions of each sub-section that represent the amount of hair to be cut at one time. When planning the partings, thought should be given to the directional angles of the cut. Thick partings are used for fine, low-density hair and thin partings are used for thick, dense hair.

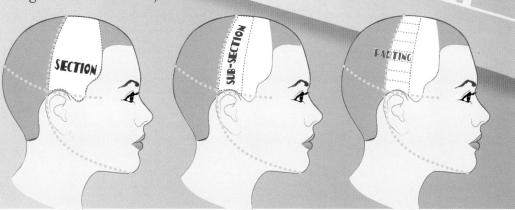

SECTION

SUB-SECTION

PARTING

Principles of Line Construction ...

In order to create the desired hairstyle, *you must first envision the shape you will be building. All shapes are created from lines: straight (horizontal, vertical and diagonal) and curved. The following principles of shape construction will help you create the shapes of haircutting:*

PRINCIPLE 1 — Points

Points can be small, medium or large.

● ● ⬤

PRINCIPLE 2 — Line Creation

Lines are created by the shifting of points, in a straight or curved direction.

PRINCIPLE 4 — Length

Lines range in length from short to long.

- **Short lines** generate a feeling of strength.
- **Long lines** generate a feeling of softness.

PRINCIPLE 5 — Line Shape

Lines are either straight or curved in shape.

- **Straight lines** represent masculinity, sport and strength.
- **Curved lines** represent femininity, gentleness and softness.

PRINCIPLE 3 — Weight

Lines can be thin or thick in weight.

- **Thin lines** provide a light feeling and appearance.
- **Thick lines** provide a heavy feeling and appearance.

PRINCIPLE 6 — Vertical Lines

Vertical lines run up and down, providing a feeling of height and depth.

1

2

HAIRCUTTING

Principles of Line Construction . . .

PRINCIPLE 7 — Horizontal Lines

Horizontal lines run side to side, providing a feeling of width.

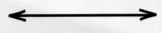

PRINCIPLE 8 — Diagonal Lines

Diagonal lines extend to opposite corners on a slant, providing counterbalance effects and a feeling of motion.

PRINCIPLE 9 — Angles

Angles are a combination of two straight lines joined together, producing various effects and qualities.

There are three basic classifications of angles:

• **Right angle:** two straight lines joined perpendicular to each other, forming a 90 degree angle.

• **Acute angle:** two straight lines joined together forming an angle less than 90 degrees.

• **Obtuse angle:** two straight lines joined together forming an angle greater than 90 degrees and less than 180 degrees.

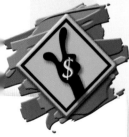

Knowledge is wealth, and great work pays off! Sell your skills by demonstrating your knowledge.

PRINCIPLE 10 — Combination Lines

The combination of straight and curved lines creates endless design element variations. The creative combination of lines will produce a blending of the characteristics of all component lines.

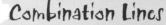

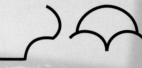

1

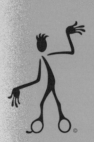

"Test your understanding of the shapes of haircutting by identifying which of the following lines are used to create the hairstyle shown."

2

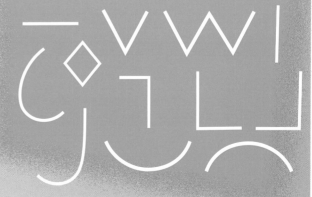

All finished haircuts can be viewed as simple, three-dimensional geometric shapes. Those three-dimensional finished shapes are created by cutting using two-dimensional lines. The haircutter views the head at a downward angle and cuts slightly below eye level. This creates the appearance of "lines" of hair that are either parallel or perpendicular to the head's surface. In reality, the lines are not actually parallel or perpendicular, because the head is a rounded surface.

By mastering the lines of haircutting, geometric hair design shapes can be created and controlled as desired for the finished cut. The lines of haircutting are categorized in the following types: **horizontal, vertical and diagonal.** Each line represents various movement and design options.

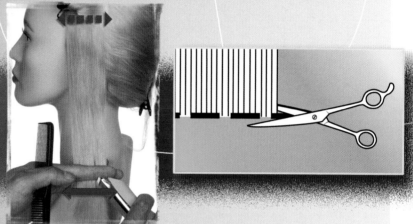

Horizontal lines create stability and weight in a haircut, without affecting directional movement. Horizontal lines can also be used as guidelines.

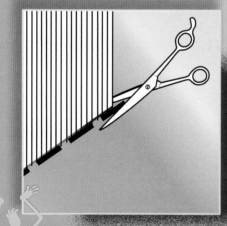

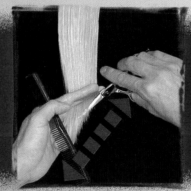

Diagonal lines create motion in a haircut by moving hair in all directions, including toward the face, away from the face or all to one side. Diagonal lines can also be used as directional guidelines.

Vertical lines are used to create the partings of a haircut. They are also used as guides for haircuts with various lengths of hair.

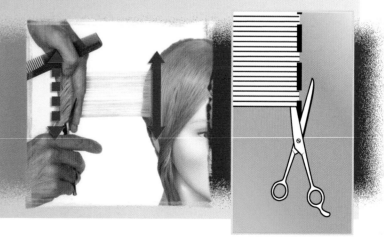

"Remember : any line can create a movement or a design pattern."

Lines ...

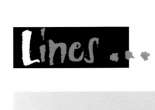

A **Vanishing** line is a line that gradually tapers off into infinity, creating an effect similar to that when viewing the parallel lines of a road disappearing in the distance.

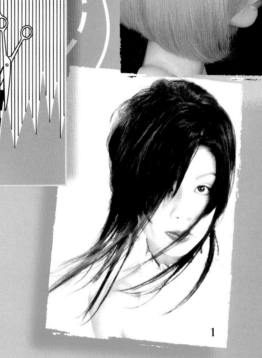

1

Curved Lines

A **curved line** *is a continuously bending line that forms part of or a complete circle. Curved lines add softness and movement to the hair.*

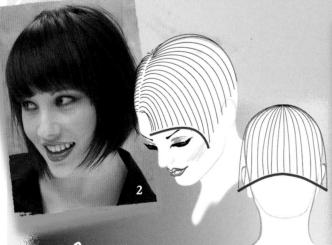

2

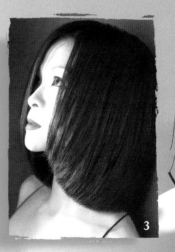

3

A **Concave** line is curved inward, in a bowl shape. The outer areas are cut longer than the inner areas.

A **Convex** line is curved outward, in an arch shape. The inner areas are cut longer than the outer areas.

Cutting Lines . . .

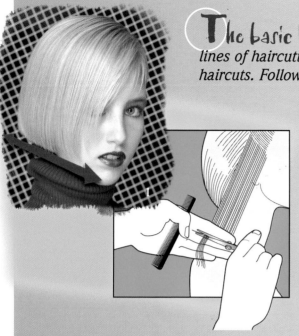

The basic lines of haircutting *form the basis for specialized lines of haircutting, which are used as guides and also to customize your haircuts. Following are some of the specialized lines of haircutting:*

Baseline:

Cutting Guide

The combination of horizontal, diagonal or curved lines creates various baselines. A baseline is the perimeter or outer boundary of a haircut. It is also referred to as a design line or a fringe line.

Guideline:

A guideline is a small section of hair used to determine the length of the next section of hair to be cut. Follow the guideline by looking through the previously cut hair section when cutting the current section.

There are two types of guidelines:

A **Stationary Guide** is a fixed or non-moving guide.
A **Traveling Guide** is a guide that moves or passes from one section to another.

STATIONARY GUIDES

TRAVELING GUIDES

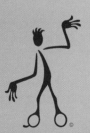

"Learn to Read The Hair. The guideline must be visible through each parting ."

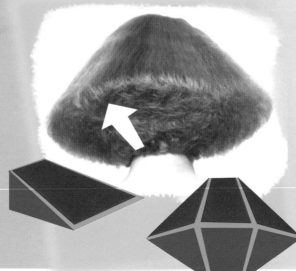

Inclination Line:

An inclination line is created by the elevation of degrees cut into the hair; for example, low to medium to high.

Head Positions ...

The position of the client's head while cutting affects the lengths of the hair. For some cuts, it is very important to keep the head in a perfectly upright, neutral position. For other cuts, tilting the head is a technique used to create elevations.

When the head is **perfectly upright** and straight, in a neutral position, the hair falls in its natural distribution.

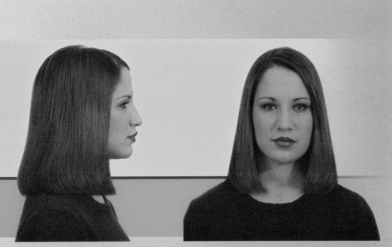

When the head is **tilted backward, forward or to either side**, elevation or graduation automatically occurs, as shown here.

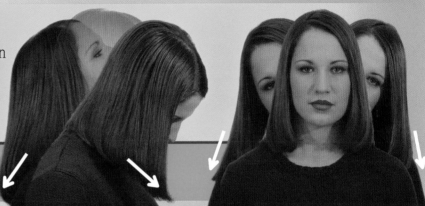

INCREASED LENGTHS are created by tilting the head forward or to the side, away from the stylist.

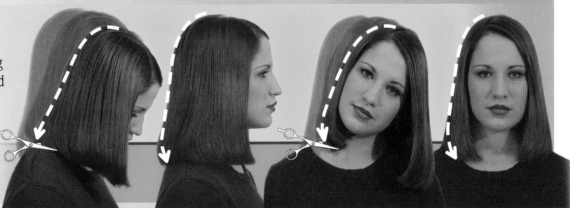

DECREASED LENGTHS are created by tilting the head backward or to the side, toward the stylist.

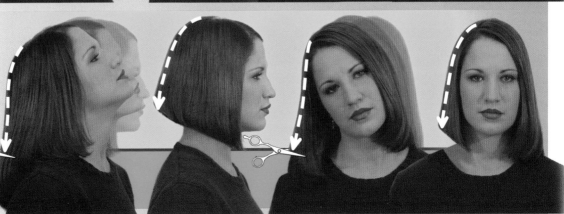

Connecting Lines . . .

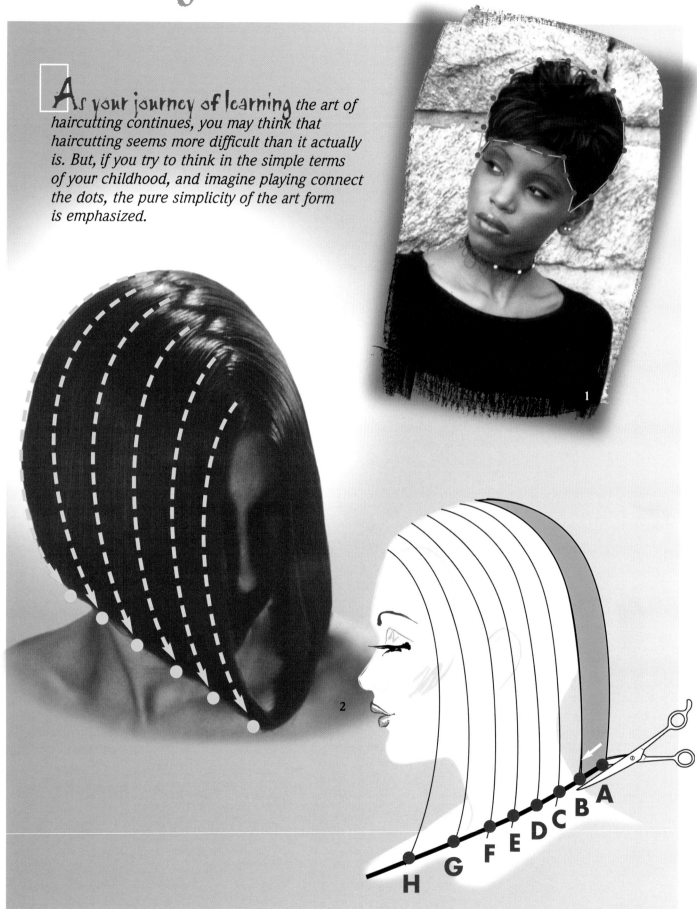

As your journey of learning the art of haircutting continues, you may think that haircutting seems more difficult than it actually is. But, if you try to think in the simple terms of your childhood, and imagine playing connect the dots, the pure simplicity of the art form is emphasized.

1

2

H G F E D C B A

HAIRCUTTING

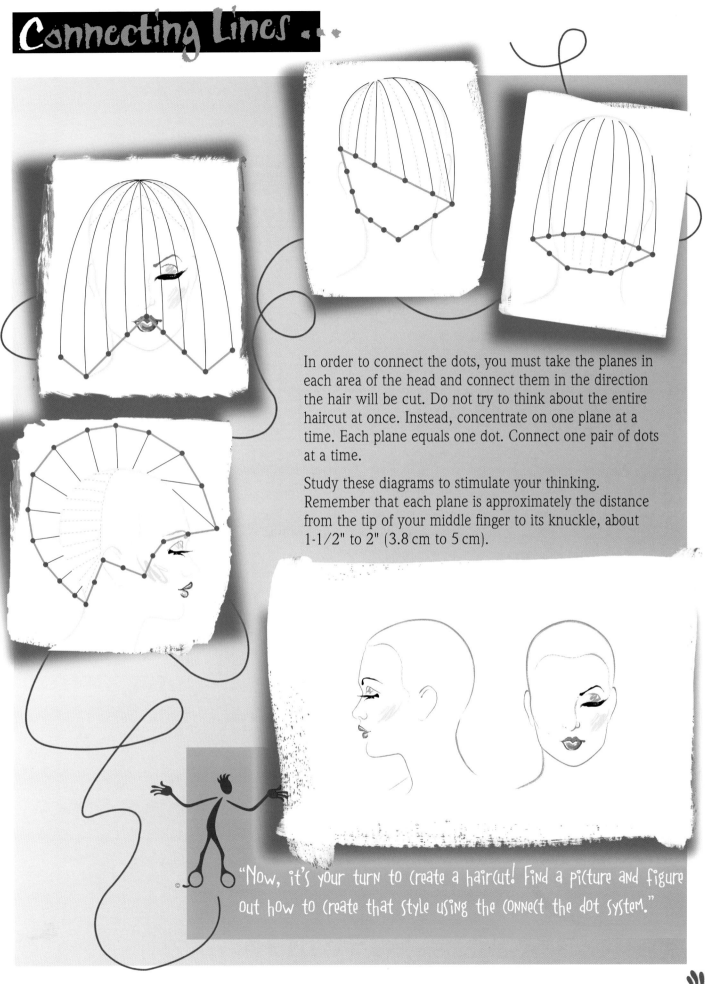

Connecting Lines

In order to connect the dots, you must take the planes in each area of the head and connect them in the direction the hair will be cut. Do not try to think about the entire haircut at once. Instead, concentrate on one plane at a time. Each plane equals one dot. Connect one pair of dots at a time.

Study these diagrams to stimulate your thinking. Remember that each plane is approximately the distance from the tip of your middle finger to its knuckle, about 1-1/2" to 2" (3.8 cm to 5 cm).

"Now, it's your turn to create a haircut! Find a picture and figure out how to create that style using the connect the dot system."

Elevations...

Elevation is created by raising hair to levels measured in degrees. *Positive and negative elevations are defined by the **degree** to which the hair is raised away from the head while cutting.*

For simplicity, the 360 degrees of a circle are reduced to the vertical and horizontal quarter panels in which the haircutter works. Each quarter panel contains the range from 0 degrees to 90 degrees.

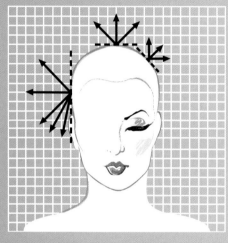

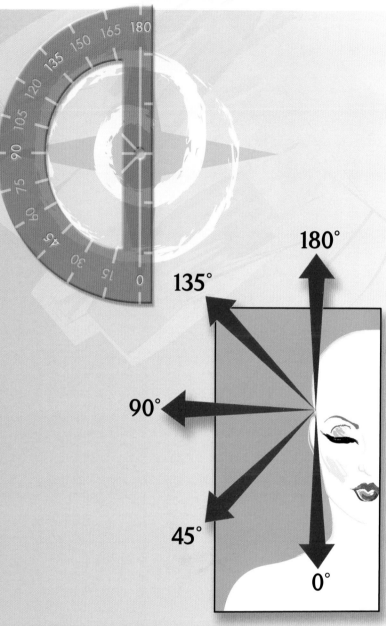

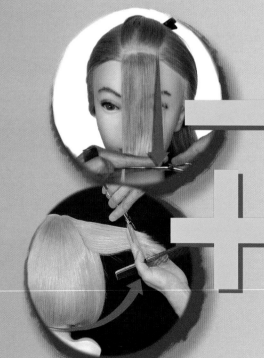

Negative elevation is created when the hair is held close to the head, at 0 degrees and then cut. Because the hair is not lifted while being cut, a concentration of lengths is created, producing weight or volume to the hairstyle.

Positive elevation is created when the hair is lifted away from the head and then cut. The levels of positive elevation cutting range from 1 degree to 180 degrees. Cutting with positive elevation creates lighter concentrations of length and mobility within the cut.

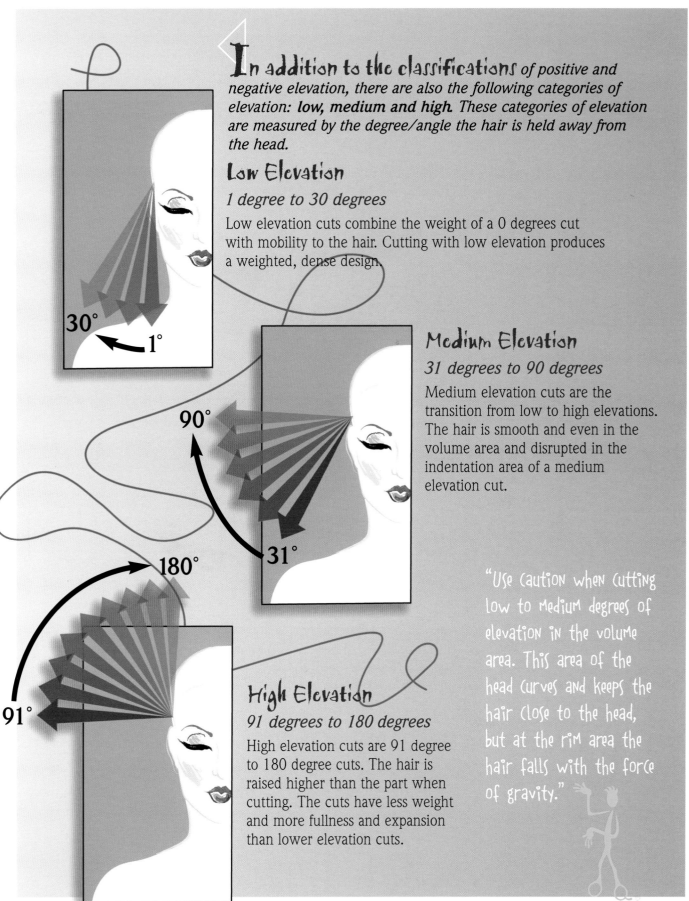

In addition to the classifications *of positive and negative elevation, there are also the following categories of elevation:* **low, medium and high.** *These categories of elevation are measured by the degree/angle the hair is held away from the head.*

Low Elevation

1 degree to 30 degrees

Low elevation cuts combine the weight of a 0 degrees cut with mobility to the hair. Cutting with low elevation produces a weighted, dense design.

30°

1°

Medium Elevation

31 degrees to 90 degrees

Medium elevation cuts are the transition from low to high elevations. The hair is smooth and even in the volume area and disrupted in the indentation area of a medium elevation cut.

90°

31°

180°

91°

High Elevation

91 degrees to 180 degrees

High elevation cuts are 91 degree to 180 degree cuts. The hair is raised higher than the part when cutting. The cuts have less weight and more fullness and expansion than lower elevation cuts.

"Use caution when cutting low to medium degrees of elevation in the volume area. This area of the head curves and keeps the hair close to the head, but at the rim area the hair falls with the force of gravity."

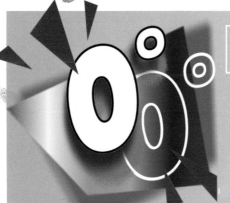

Zero degree haircuts are negative elevation cuts (also known as blunt, one-length and compact), requiring no lifting or raising of the hair during the cutting process. The hair lengths are concentrated in a single line when the hair is in its natural distribution. This concentration of lengths gives width to the cut, creating the appearance of volume and weight. Although 0 degree cuts appear to be one length, **the actual hair length in the indentation area is shorter than in the volume area.** The finished texture is smooth and continuous, since there are no broken lines within the haircut.

negative
blunt
one length
compact

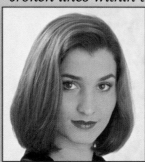
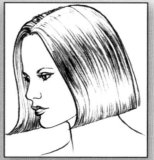
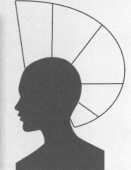

Following are basic principles of 0 degree haircuts:

- **Stationary Guideline.** All partings are released and brought down to the guideline.
- **Maintain Natural Distribution.** Create the appearance of a single line by maintaining a natural distribution of hair over the curve of the head.
- **Partings Parallel to Guideline.** Partings should be parallel to the intended base or guideline at all times.
- **Scissors and Fingers Parallel to Guideline.** Scissors and finger positions should remain parallel to the intended base or guideline at all times.
- **Hair Flat to Head.** The hand position must be against the head and the hair combed flat to the head to maintain 0 degrees.

The following factors will influence the quality of finished 0 degree haircuts:

- **Client Head Position.** Adjusting the client's head position influences how the hair travels over the curve of the head. The optimal cutting position is when the head is straight, causing the hair to fall naturally over the curve, producing a single line. Don't position the head forward, because the hair travels farther to reach the guideline and therefore the top layers are cut longer than the underneath layers.
- **Tension/Pressure.** Applying tension or pressure stretches the hair prior to cutting. When the tension is released, the hair contracts, creating the appearance of shorter lengths and volume. Be sure to allow for tension when cutting textures such as curly hair, to prevent the end result from being too short.
- **Hand Position.** Use a palm upward position (palm to palm) to create a small amount of elevation, giving the hair some mobility.
- **Distribution.** Don't shift the hair in any direction but its natural distribution over the curve of the head, to avoid variation in the lengths of the finished cut.
- **Texture.** Natural curl or wave automatically creates small degrees of elevation within the cut.

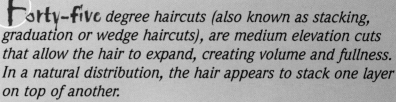

Degrees of Cutting...

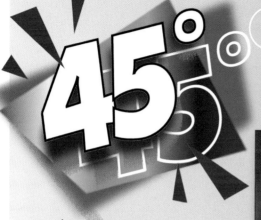

45°

stacking
graduation
wedge

Forty-five degree haircuts (also known as stacking, graduation or wedge haircuts), are medium elevation cuts that allow the hair to expand, creating volume and fullness. In a natural distribution, the hair appears to stack one layer on top of another.

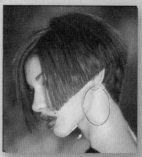 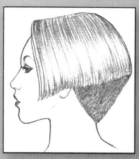 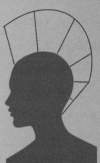

Following are basic principles of 45 degree haircuts:

- **Positive Projection.** Positive projection is used to cut the various degrees of elevation.
- **Stationary and Traveling Guidelines.** Either type of guideline can be used.
- **Vertical Parting Pattern.** Any parting pattern can be used. Remember to keep the fingers and scissors parallel. The angle of your finger in relation to the curve of the client's head will influence the degree of elevation.
- **Hair Distribution.** The distribution of the hair over the head influences the elevation. Hair in its natural distribution requires lifting to create elevation. Shifting of the hair creates elevation without lifting.
- **Palm Upward Position.** Use a palm upward position (palm to palm) to elevate the hair. The guide is visible, and therefore clean, and precise lines are created.
- **Head Position.** The head position should be upright except when cutting below the weight line.

The following factors will influence the quality of finished 45 degree haircuts:

- **Combining Techniques.** Using various techniques in combination will customize the finished cut. For example, applying tension/pressure and shifting the hair from its natural distribution will increase the degree of elevation.
- **Natural Hair Texture.** Curled hair texture creates a natural lift. When elevation is applied to the cut it will intensify the finished result.

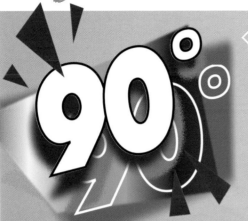

Ninety degree haircuts are positive elevation cuts with the hair lifted 90 degrees during cutting. When the entire head is uniformly cut at 90 degrees, all lengths are exactly the same, whether in a natural distribution or projected state. These uniform lengths do not provide weight to the cut, but do provide mobility. *Vertical, horizontal* or *diagonal finger positions* will create a 90-degree haircut–staying parallel to parting; any deviation from 90 degrees while cutting will produce uneven lengths. The texture of the hair is completely layered, following the contour of the head.

radial

brush cut

layered cut

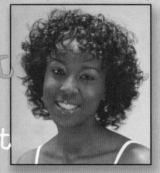
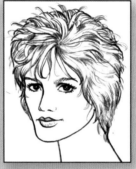
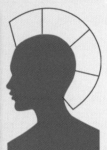

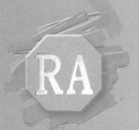

Following are basic principles of 90 degree haircuts:

- **Traveling Guide.** A traveling guide, consisting of small amounts of previously cut hair, is used as the guide for each new parting.
- **Equal Lengths and Projection.** Lengths are projected straight out from the head at 90 degrees during cutting. Lengths are constant and equal, with visible ends.
- **Palm Upward Position.** When working in the volume area, the palm faces upward and cutting is on top of the hand. In the indentation area, the palm faces either upward or outward, depending upon the curve of the head and if you are cutting vertically, horizontally or diagonally.
- **Any Parting Pattern.** Horizontal, vertical or diagonal parting patterns can be used. For vertical parts, the fingers must remain parallel to the curve of the head.
- **Palm Upward or Downward.** Depending upon the area of the head being cut, a palm upward or downward position can be used.

The following factors will influence the quality of finished 90 degree haircuts:

- **Deviation from 90 degrees.** Any deviation from 90 degree elevation will create increased or decreased lengths.
- **Finger Position.** Any increase or decrease in finger position will create increased or decreased lengths.
- **Head Position.** The head should be in a natural upright position to create uniform layers of 90 degrees.

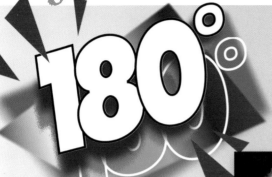

Degrees of Cutting . . .

long layers
reverse
increase

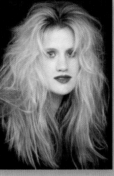
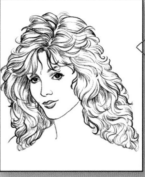
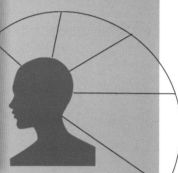

One hundred eighty degree cuts feature shorter lengths in the volume area progressing to longer lengths in the indentation area. Minimum to no weight is present in the cut. In a natural distribution the ends are exposed, adding movement and diversity.

Following are basic principles of 180 degree haircuts:

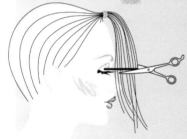

- **Positive or Negative Elevation.** Either positive or negative elevation can be used in the volume area to create a layered appearance.
- **Squeeze Cutting.** In a squeeze cutting technique, all hair is gathered to a single degree and then cut. This is called an "automatic graduation." Each strand of hair travels a different distance to reach that degree, therefore creating various lengths with a single cutting process. Refer to page 114.
- **Stationary Guideline.** All lengths are directed to a stationary guideline for squeeze cutting. As the hair travels across the curve of the head, layers are created. (Note: When a traveling guideline is used to create this cut, finger position and distribution of hair are critical factors. Fingers must extend outward from the curve of the head and lengths are shifted to that guide).
- **Parting Pattern.** Horizontal partings are recommended.
- **Direct Hair in Opposite Direction.** Direct the hair in the direction opposite from the desired movement. For example, if you want to move the hair toward the face, direct it backwards to the control area of the head for cutting.

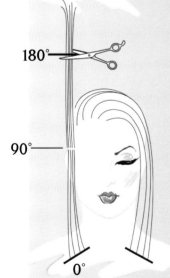

The following factors will influence the quality of finished 180 degree haircuts:

- **Head Position.** If the head is positioned downward, the hair must travel farther to reach the guideline, thereby creating longer length in the indentation area.
- **Finger Position.** If the fingers are in any position other than parallel, the lengths will either be decreased or increased. For example, when working in the front hairline area and positioning the fingers outward at an angle away from the face, lengths will increase.

Chapter 4 • **MATHEMATICS OF HAIRCUTTING** 113

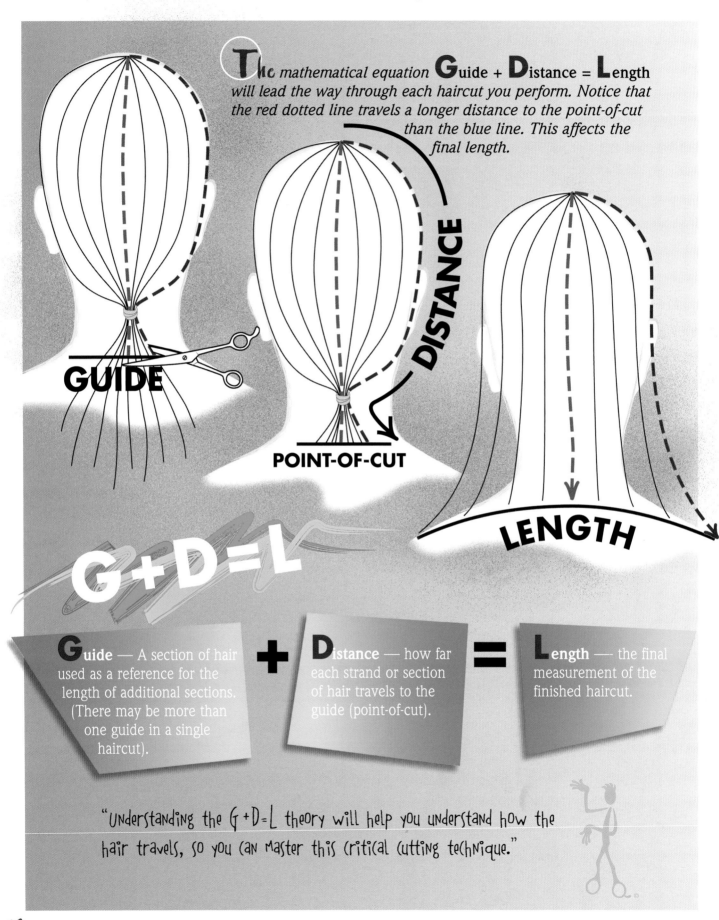

The mathematical equation **G**uide + **D**istance = **L**ength will lead the way through each haircut you perform. Notice that the red dotted line travels a longer distance to the point-of-cut than the blue line. This affects the final length.

GUIDE

DISTANCE

POINT-OF-CUT

LENGTH

G+D=L

Guide — A section of hair used as a reference for the length of additional sections. (There may be more than one guide in a single haircut).

+

Distance — how far each strand or section of hair travels to the guide (point-of-cut).

=

Length — the final measurement of the finished haircut.

"Understanding the G+D=L theory will help you understand how the hair travels, so you can master this critical cutting technique."

Guide + Distance = Length ...

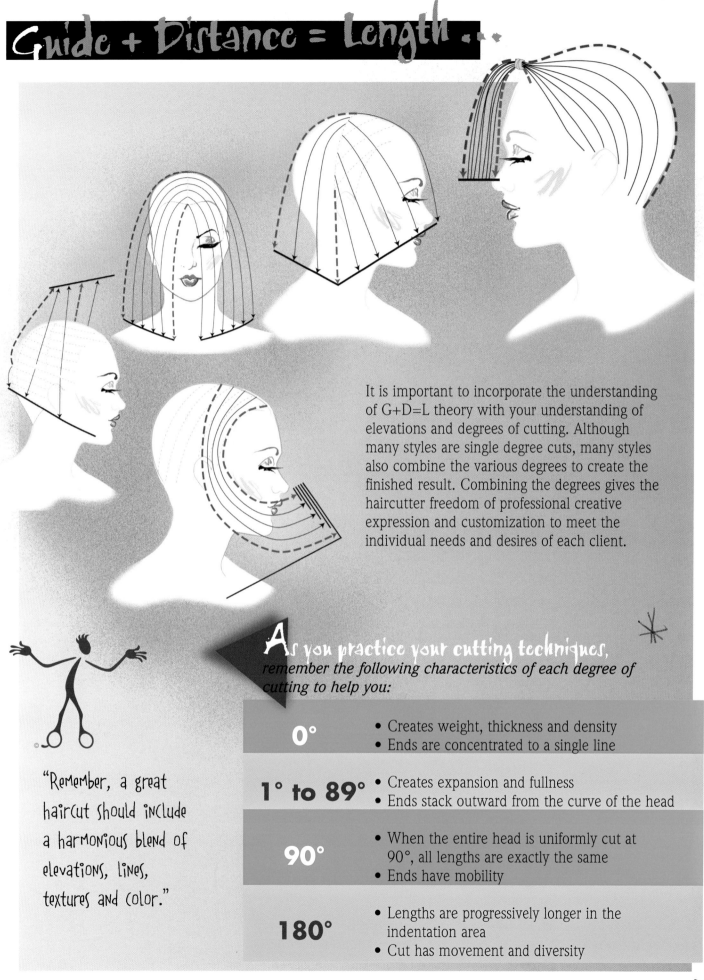

It is important to incorporate the understanding of G+D=L theory with your understanding of elevations and degrees of cutting. Although many styles are single degree cuts, many styles also combine the various degrees to create the finished result. Combining the degrees gives the haircutter freedom of professional creative expression and customization to meet the individual needs and desires of each client.

As you practice your cutting techniques, remember the following characteristics of each degree of cutting to help you:

0°	• Creates weight, thickness and density • Ends are concentrated to a single line
1° to 89°	• Creates expansion and fullness • Ends stack outward from the curve of the head
90°	• When the entire head is uniformly cut at 90°, all lengths are exactly the same • Ends have mobility
180°	• Lengths are progressively longer in the indentation area • Cut has movement and diversity

"Remember, a great haircut should include a harmonious blend of elevations, lines, textures and color."

Harmonic Progression...

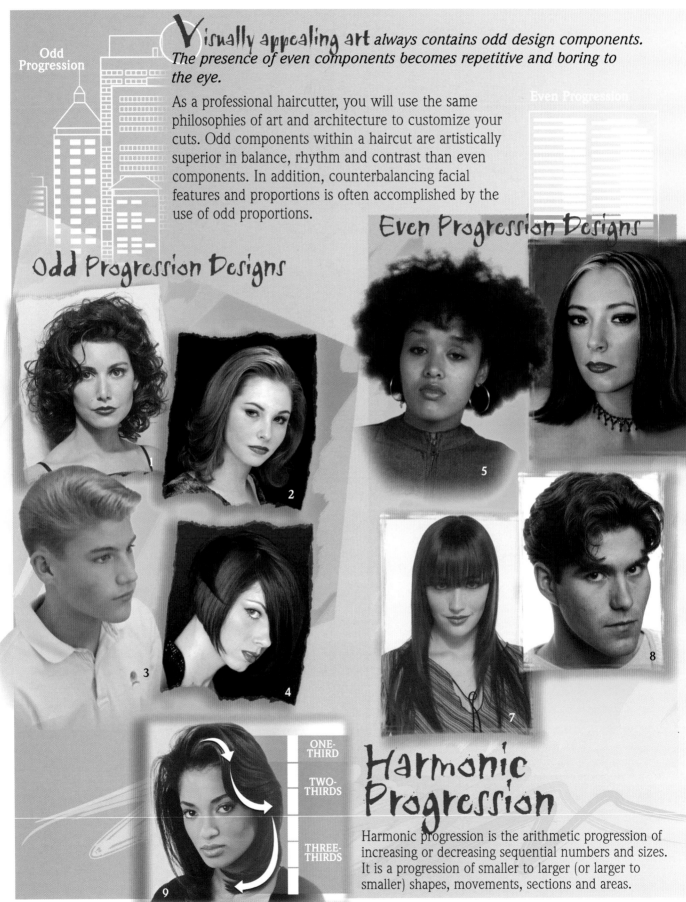

Visually appealing art *always contains odd design components. The presence of even components becomes repetitive and boring to the eye.*

As a professional haircutter, you will use the same philosophies of art and architecture to customize your cuts. Odd components within a haircut are artistically superior in balance, rhythm and contrast than even components. In addition, counterbalancing facial features and proportions is often accomplished by the use of odd proportions.

Odd Progression

Even Progression

Odd Progression Designs

Even Progression Designs

Harmonic Progression

Harmonic progression is the arithmetic progression of increasing or decreasing sequential numbers and sizes. It is a progression of smaller to larger (or larger to smaller) shapes, movements, sections and areas.

ONE-THIRD

TWO-THIRDS

THREE-THIRDS

Unbalanced Progression ...

When the design elements progress in an unbalanced manner, disproportionate rhythms, weights, textures and speeds emerge. Usually found in haircuts without any blending or transitioning, unbalanced progressions occur in many forms. The following examples illustrate this concept:

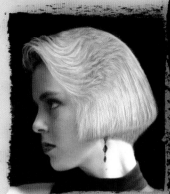

Better

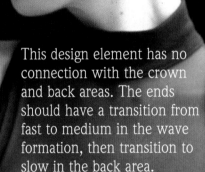

2

This design element has no connection with the crown and back areas. The ends should have a transition from fast to medium in the wave formation, then transition to slow in the back area.

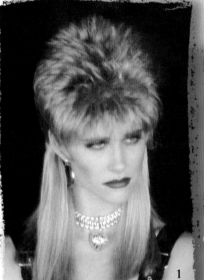

1

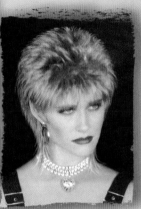

Better

This haircut design gives the appearance of two different haircuts—a short 90 degree haircut in front and a 0 degree haircut in the back. The two different textures also over-emphasize the different haircuts.

"Remember to blend the frontal, crown and occipital areas of the head to connect the design elements of each component in harmonious progression."

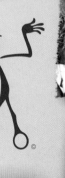

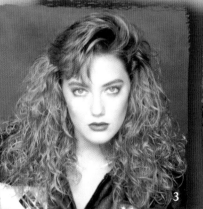

3

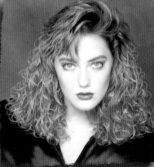

Better

The hair in this design is separated in texture and length and therefore does not show proper proportions. The hanging lengths should be shorter to help minimize the two textures.

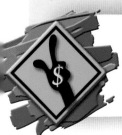

Promoting the magic of makeovers is a wonderful way to sell your services while helping your clients look their best!

The Seven Steps of Haircutting...

By following a standard sequence of steps for each haircut, you will ensure quality and consistency of the finished results of your work. Let's review the seven steps of precision haircutting.

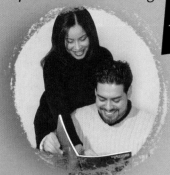

1. Client Consultation

Before every haircut (even on repeat customers) it is important to consult with clients about the results they desire. Listening and reinforcing your understanding of what is requested is the most important element of effective communication. During the consultation, you have an opportunity to evaluate the client's lifestyle, facial features and body proportions as you begin to conceptualize and visualize the optimal cut.

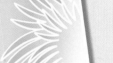

Always discuss prices prior to your services, to avoid surprises for your client.

2. Hair Analysis

Evaluate the hair of each client to help determine the components of the haircut and style that will create the best end results. The following elements should be considered:

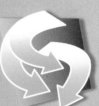

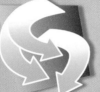

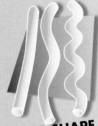

TEXTURE.
Textural elements of the hair will either need to be enhanced or minimized to complement the final cut.

DENSITY.
Hair density is used to create volume. It is difficult to achieve volume in areas where hair is sparse. Common areas of thinness include the crown, around the ears, the fringe area and the nape.

GROWTH PATTERN.
Determining growth patterns is the blueprint of hair movement, and therefore will influence design decisions. Hair length, cutting tension, and degrees of elevation are all influenced by growth patterns.

HAIR SHAPE.
The shape of the hair (straight, wavy or curly) determines whether it should be cut wet or dry, how short it should be cut, and the customizing techniques needed to enhance the cut.

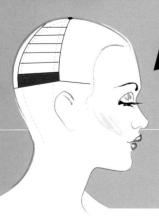

3. Sectioning

Never include more hair in a section than you can control. Appropriate sectioning and parting of the hair provides the quality control for the haircut. It is also the blueprint to follow to create the elevations of the cut.

4. Baseline

The baseline is the frame that forms the bottom outer perimeter of the haircut. Development of the baseline provides a reference guide for the entire cut, which can include many lines and textures. Remember, more than one guide can exist in each haircut.

The Seven Steps of Haircutting...

5. Distribution and Elevation

Accurately project the hair to the desired elevation, keeping the following elements in mind:

DISTRIBUTION DIRECTIONS
- **Natural:** Hair is distributed over the head in the natural growth pattern.
- **Shifted:** Hair is distributed in any direction other than natural. Different elevations are automatically created by shifting.

POSITIVE OR NEGATIVE ELEVATION
Examine the client's hair for density, growth direction and texture. Also, determine the length necessary for the desired style. These elements will determine how much each area should be elevated to build weight or create lightness in the finished haircut.

DEGREES
Calculate the degrees needed for your architectural haircut design. Then precision cut each component of the style by the degree or combination of degrees needed to achieve a strong foundation to support the finished hairdesign.

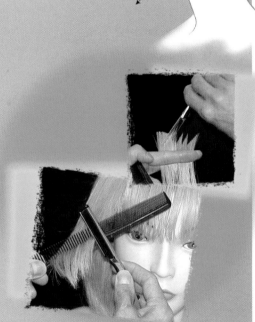

6. Customizing

After the form of the haircut has been established, many different customizing tools and techniques can be used to personalize the cut for current fashions and styles. Primary areas of the hair strand which are customized include the scalp, center and ends. Refer to Chapter 5.

7. Check

The final step of each haircut is checking. **Cross-checking** at the end of haircut is subsectioning the hair the opposite way from the actual haircut using the same degree as the cut. This is a critical concluding step, because it verifies the precision and accuracy of the completed cut. Always criss-cross your cut to ensure a perfect blend of lengths. Clean the baseline to adjust any undesirable, irregular lengths.

Don't forget the 3 R's at the end of every service.

RETAIL • RE-BOOK • REFERRAL

The development of a haircut design involves a series of decisions that influence other elements of the cut down the line. This quick reference guide presents a visual overview of the flow of decision making when performing a haircut.

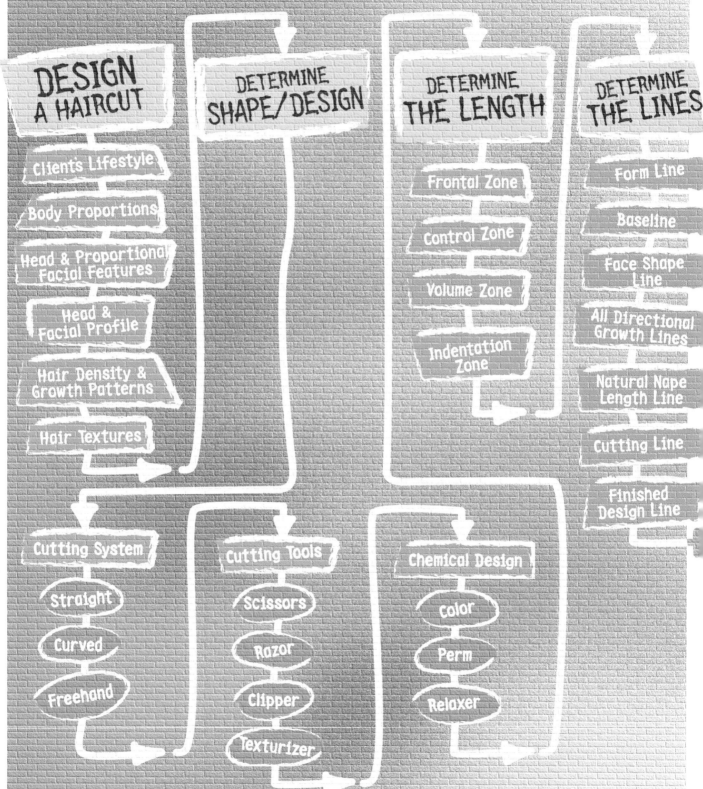

DESIGN A HAIRCUT
- Clients Lifestyle
- Body Proportions
- Head & Proportional Facial Features
- Head & Facial Profile
- Hair Density & Growth Patterns
- Hair Textures

DETERMINE SHAPE/DESIGN

DETERMINE THE LENGTH
- Frontal Zone
- Control Zone
- Volume Zone
- Indentation Zone

DETERMINE THE LINES
- Form Line
- Baseline
- Face Shape Line
- All Directional Growth Lines
- Natural Nape Length Line
- Cutting Line
- Finished Design Line

Cutting System
- Straight
- Curved
- Freehand

Cutting Tools
- Scissors
- Razor
- Clipper
- Texturizer

Chemical Design
- Color
- Perm
- Relaxer

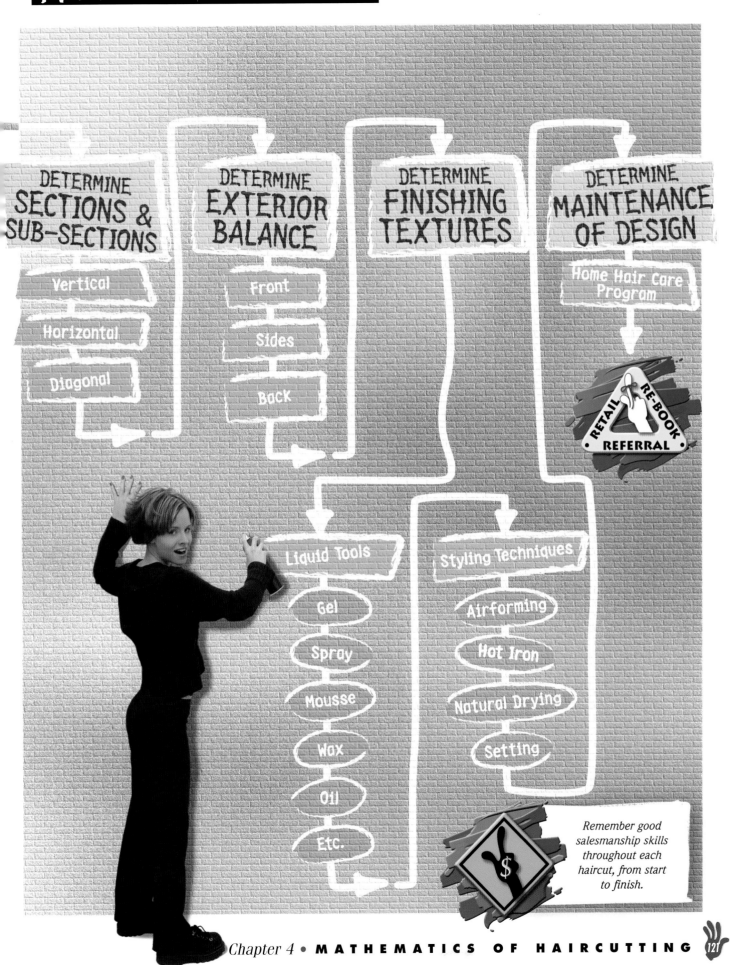

Haircut Flow Chart ... Quick Reference Guide

DETERMINE SECTIONS & SUB-SECTIONS
- Vertical
- Horizontal
- Diagonal

DETERMINE EXTERIOR BALANCE
- Front
- Sides
- Back

DETERMINE FINISHING TEXTURES

DETERMINE MAINTENANCE OF DESIGN
- Home Hair Care Program

RETAIL · RE-BOOK · REFERRAL

Liquid Tools
- Gel
- Spray
- Mousse
- Wax
- Oil
- Etc.

Styling Techniques
- Airforming
- Hot Iron
- Natural Drying
- Setting

Remember good salesmanship skills throughout each haircut, from start to finish.

Chapter 4 • **MATHEMATICS OF HAIRCUTTING**

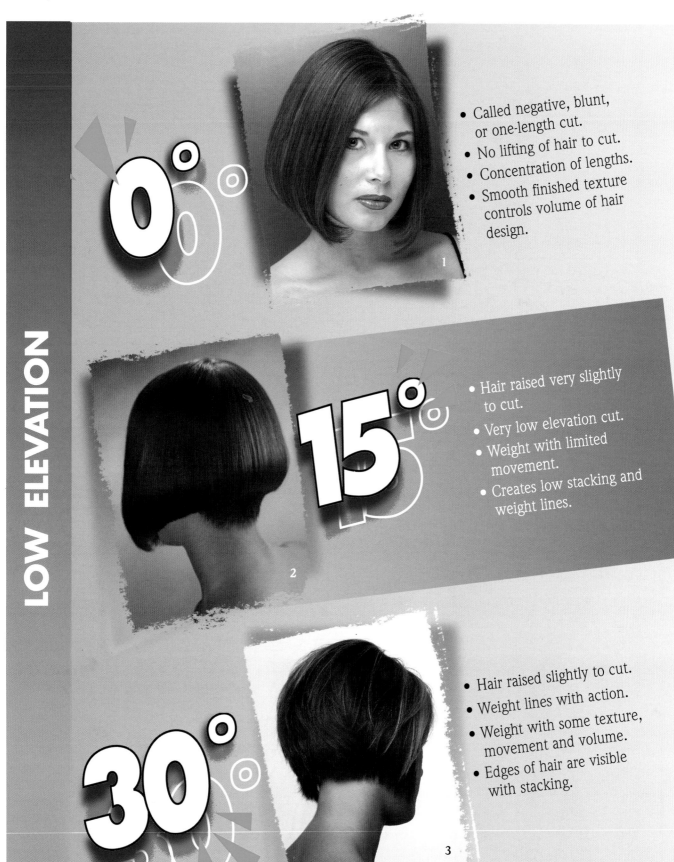

LOW ELEVATION

0°

- Called negative, blunt, or one-length cut.
- No lifting of hair to cut.
- Concentration of lengths.
- Smooth finished texture controls volume of hair design.

1

15°

- Hair raised very slightly to cut.
- Very low elevation cut.
- Weight with limited movement.
- Creates low stacking and weight lines.

2

30°

- Hair raised slightly to cut.
- Weight lines with action.
- Weight with some texture, movement and volume.
- Edges of hair are visible with stacking.

3

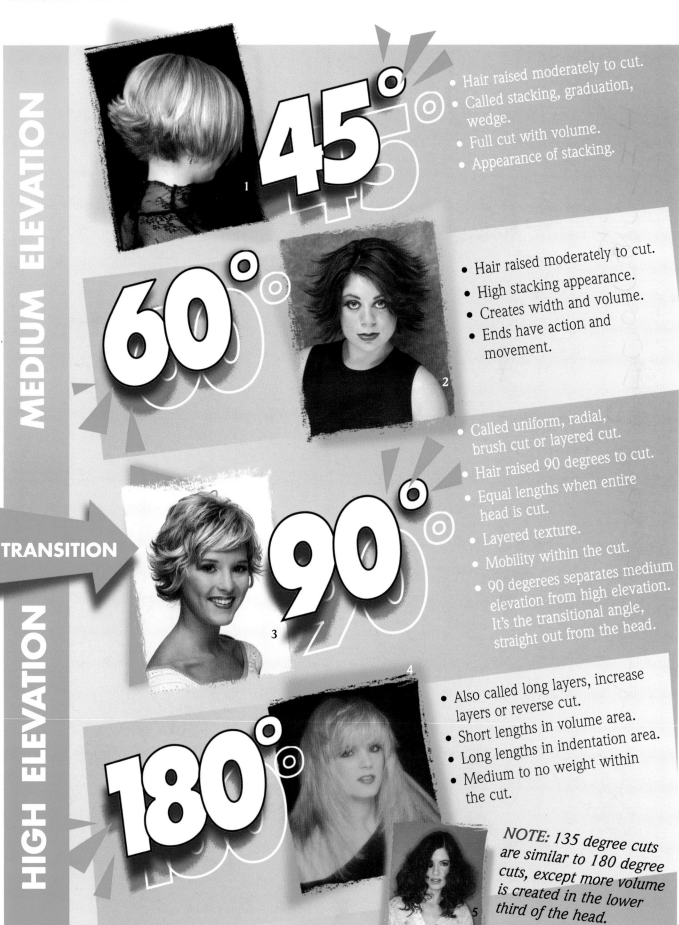

Elevations ...

MEDIUM ELEVATION

45°

- Hair raised moderately to cut.
- Called stacking, graduation, wedge.
- Full cut with volume.
- Appearance of stacking.

1

60°

- Hair raised moderately to cut.
- High stacking appearance.
- Creates width and volume.
- Ends have action and movement.

2

TRANSITION

HIGH ELEVATION

90°

- Called uniform, radial, brush cut or layered cut.
- Hair raised 90 degrees to cut.
- Equal lengths when entire head is cut.
- Layered texture.
- Mobility within the cut.
- 90 degerees separates medium elevation from high elevation. It's the transitional angle, straight out from the head.

3

180°

- Also called long layers, increase layers or reverse cut.
- Short lengths in volume area.
- Long lengths in indentation area.
- Medium to no weight within the cut.

4

NOTE: 135 degree cuts are similar to 180 degree cuts, except more volume is created in the lower third of the head.

5

Divisions of the Head

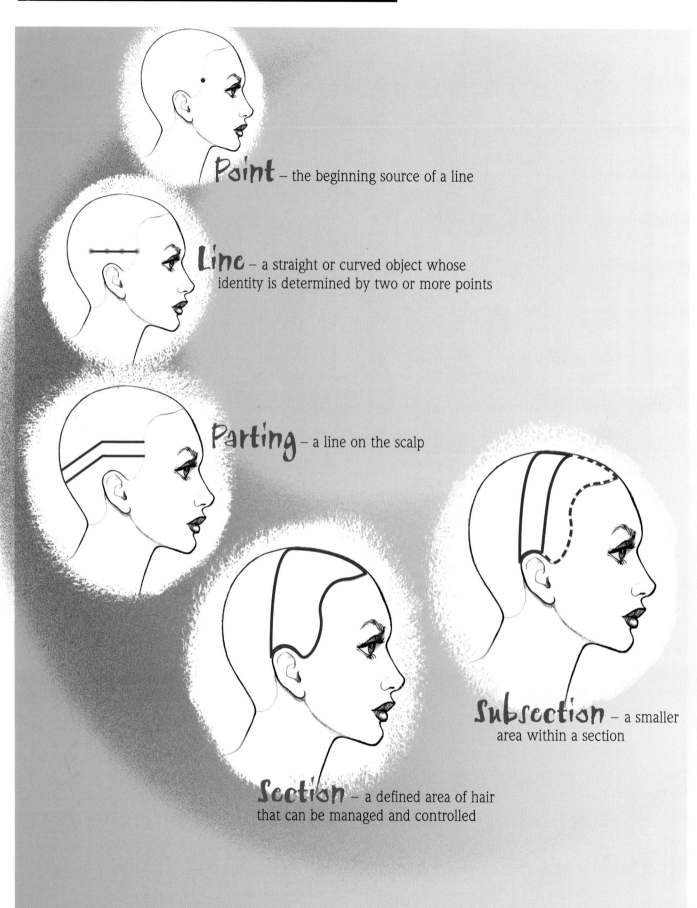

Point – the beginning source of a line

Line – a straight or curved object whose identity is determined by two or more points

Parting – a line on the scalp

Subsection – a smaller area within a section

Section – a defined area of hair that can be managed and controlled

"There are different methods of dividing the head to achieve the various objectives of each haircut. This guide is a helpful overview of the major divisions of the head — all in one handy location!"

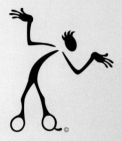

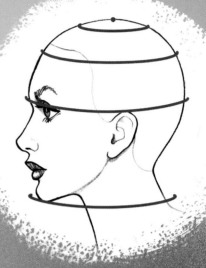

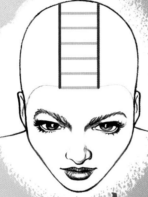

Zones – areas that encircle the head and are used as a reference for balancing and counterbalancing

Boundaries – the partings (lines) that separate the planes of the head

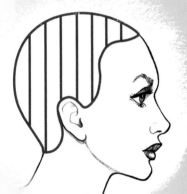

Plane – a flat area on a curved surface

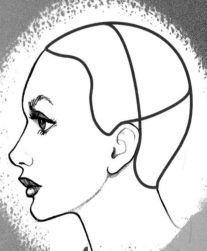

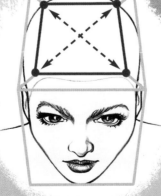

Corners – the four points on the top of the head that define the widest part of the fringe area and the widest part of the crown area

Areas – the three main components for haircutting: frontal, crown and occipital

The blueprint for creating each haircut consists of the sections and partings of the cut. Just as an architect has creative freedom when developing blue-prints, the haircutter also has freedom of artistic judgment and expression when creating sec-tions and partings.

It is exciting to have complete creative freedom and judgment, but it is also important to understand the fundamentals of sectioning and parting to guide your judgment for the best finished results.

"In the beginning stages of learning to cut, the sections and partings will be provided for you. As you progress and develop your skills, you can begin to use your knowledge of correct parting placement."

Guidelines for Sectioning and Parting:

• Consider the basic shape of the haircut as you evaluate the density, growth patterns and textures of the hair.
• Make partings thinner on thick density hair and thicker on thin density hair.
• Make partings parallel to the cutting line or guideline.

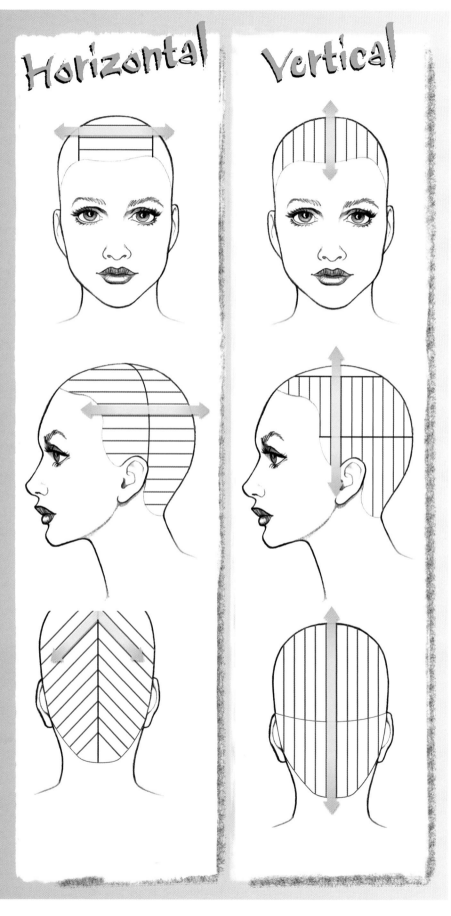

Horizontal

Vertical

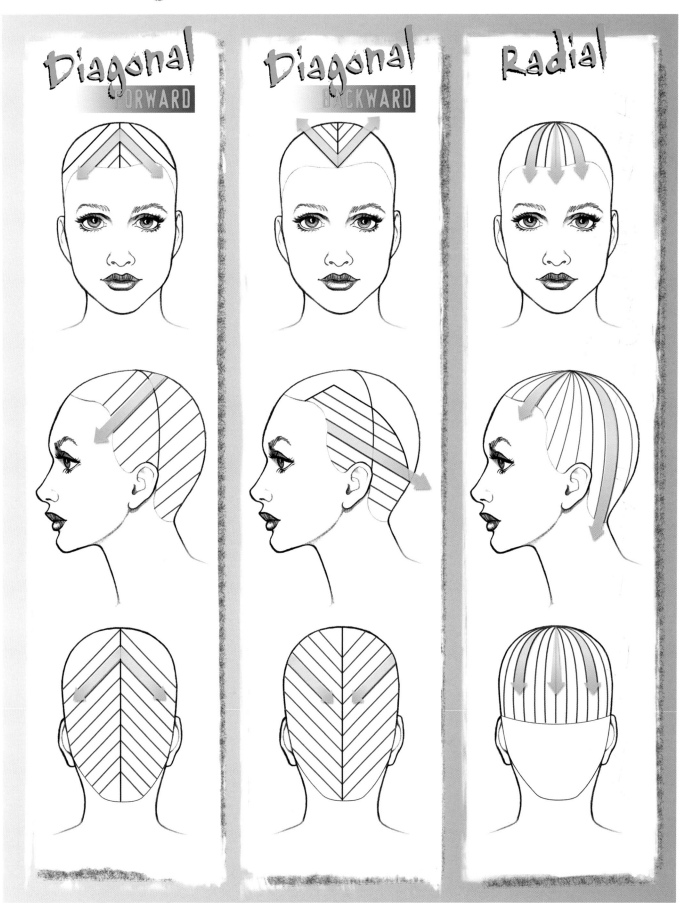

Diagonal FORWARD

Diagonal BACKWARD

Radial

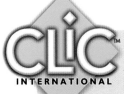

MATCHING

_I_ **1.** Lines that create motion in a haircut.   **A.** Draft

_H_ **2.** Known as a wedge or stacked cut.   **B.** Concave

_F_ **3.** Weighted, dense haircuts.   **C.** Checking

_E_ **4.** Lines that curve outward.   **D.** Guidelines

_J_ **5.** Transition from medium to high elevation.   **E.** Convex

_C_ **6.** The final step of each haircut.   **F.** Low elevation

_B_ **7.** Lines that curve inward.   **G.** High elevation

_G_ **8.** Lightweight cuts, with fullness.   **H.** 45 degree

_A_ **9.** 2-dimensional "wet-sketch."   **I.** Diagonal

_D_ **10.** Stationary and traveling.   **J.** 90 degree

TRUE OR FALSE:

_F_ **1.** The three main components for haircutting are the nape, crown and fringe areas.

_T_ **2.** Larger partings are used for fine hair and smaller partings are used for thick hair.

_T_ **3.** Lines are created by the shifting of points, either in a straight or curved direction.

_F_ **4.** The position of the client's head while cutting doesn't affect the lengths of the hair.

_T_ **5.** G+D=L explains how the hair travels different distances to the point of cut and affects the final lengths.

_F_ **6.** Visually appealing art always contains ~~even~~ _odd_ design components.

_T_ **7.** Hair analysis prior to the cut should include examination of density, growth patterns, hair shape and texture.

_F_ **8.** Customizing techniques are done at the beginning of the cut.

_T_ **9.** Partings should always be parallel to the guide line or cutting line.

_T_ **10.** Connecting the dots is a simple way to understand the planes of haircutting.

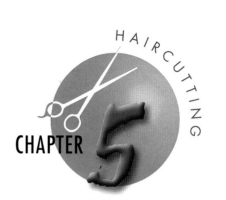

dexterity **customizing**

positioning

texturizing

parallels

planes

disruption

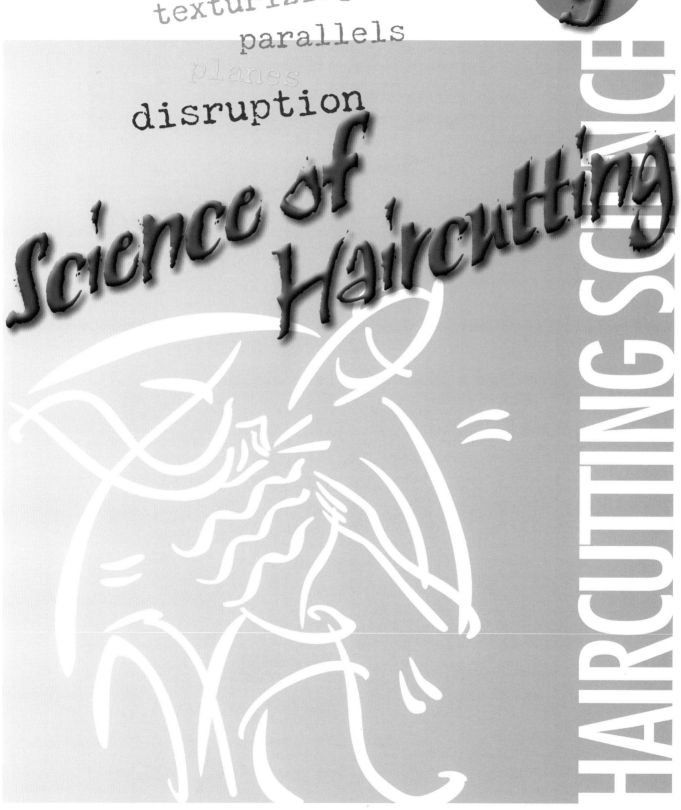

Science of Haircutting

HAIRCUTTING SCIENCE

Problem Solving...

"How do we know everything we know about life? Did you ever really stop to think about it? The scientific method is a valuable method for problem solving in everyday life, not just in the science lab."

The Scientific Method *of problem solving is a standard procedure used to evaluate criteria and develop accurate theories to explain and predict future events. By following the steps of the scientific method to develop answers, any existing perceptions or beliefs are replaced by tested and proven theories.*

Following are the 4 steps of the scientific method:

1 Identify the Problem.
Observe and describe an incident or event. This occurs when a problem or question is first identified.

2 Develop an Explanation.
Develop a hypothesis to explain the incident or event. The hypothesis is a tentative assumption about what is causing the incident or event.

3 Predict Future Events.
Use the hypothesis to predict other incidents or events. If the assumptions are correct, then future incidents or events should be able to be predicted based on the assumptions.

4 Test Predictions.
Perform experimental tests of the predictions. If the tests prove the predictions are true, then the hypothesis is accepted as a theory or law of nature. If the tests do not prove the predictions, then steps two through four must be modified and repeated until proven accurate.

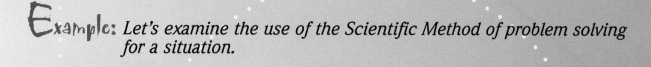

Problem Solving...

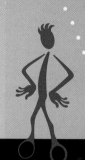

Example: *Let's examine the use of the Scientific Method of problem solving for a situation.*

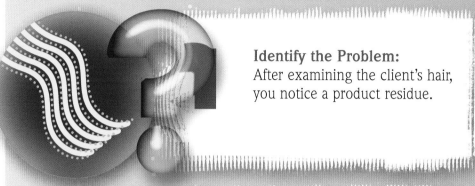

Identify the Problem:
After examining the client's hair, you notice a product residue.

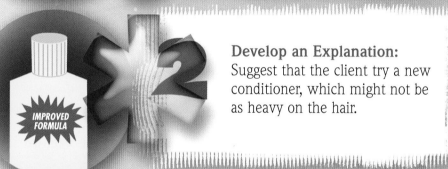

Develop an Explanation:
Suggest that the client try a new conditioner, which might not be as heavy on the hair.

Predict Future Events:
Explain that the use of a recommended professional conditioner will create a light, shiny finish to the hair.

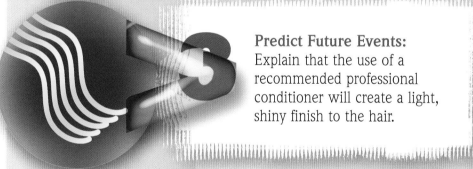

"By following a systematic approach, future events can be predicted. This is important to remember as you learn the systematic approach to cutting hair. Following this approach will allow you to deliver consistent cuts every time."

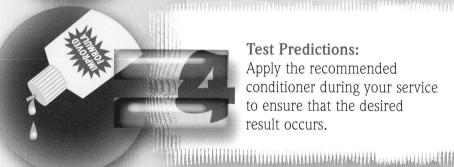

Test Predictions:
Apply the recommended conditioner during your service to ensure that the desired result occurs.

By solving your clients' problems, you help create a satisfied customer who will rebook, refer and purchase your professional retail products.

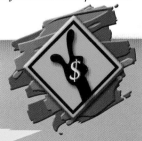

The Circle ...

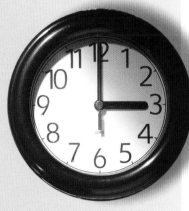

The Circular Shape

Picture a circle in your mind, or find a circular shape (such as a round clock or watch face) to look at. What do you see?

The CLiC Cutting Concept (C.C.C.) is based upon the mathematical theory of a circle, which dates back thousands of years to the time of the ancient Babylonians. The C.C.C. Theory has completed the full cycle of the scientific method and is therefore accepted as the optimal approach to haircutting. Let's examine the components of the CCC Theory.

The Degrees of a Circle

Now, look at the circle diagram below. The circle can be divided into 360 equal, angular units called degrees. If a series of tangent lines are drawn around the circle, touching each of the 360 degree points, you will discover that a circular shape is formed by the connection of angular straight lines tangent to the 360 degree points of a circle.

A **tangent line** touches a curved surface at a single point.

Our eyes interpret the angular connection of lines at the degree points as one continuous curve.

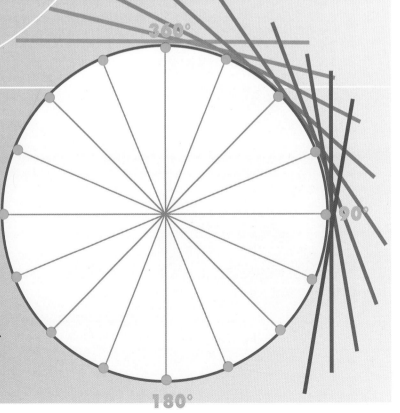

The Cutting Planes of the Head . . .

Finding The Cutting Planes

To find a plane (straight area) on the head (curved surface), follow these simple steps:

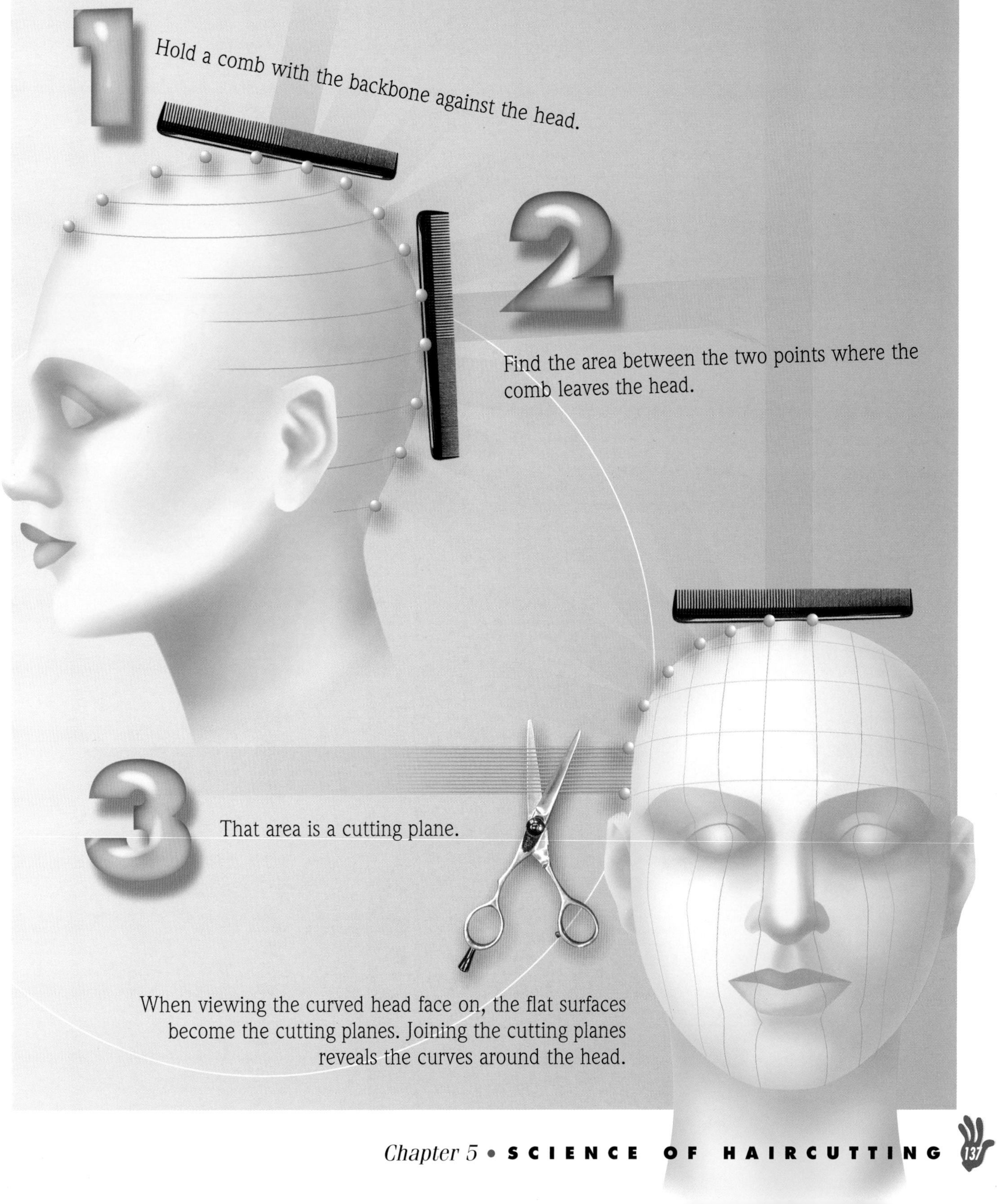

1 Hold a comb with the backbone against the head.

2 Find the area between the two points where the comb leaves the head.

3 That area is a cutting plane.

When viewing the curved head face on, the flat surfaces become the cutting planes. Joining the cutting planes reveals the curves around the head.

The combination of **The Law, The Skill and The Parallels** creates cutting perfection. Let's examine each component of perfect cutting:

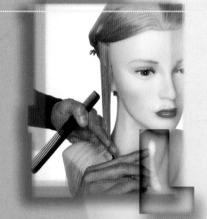

The Law

With the **C.C.C. Theory** as your foundation, you will master the LAW of cutting and have confidence to cut all textures of hair.

any *angles* to the hair

any type of *weight* into the hair

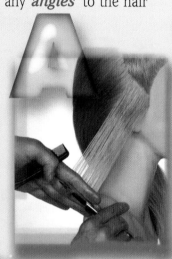

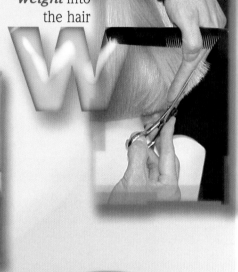

any *length* of hair

The Skill

Mastery of the **C.C.C. Theory** involves a combination of dexterity, knowledge and discipline.

Knowledge
Understanding the basic features and proper use of cutting tools is a prerequisite to success.

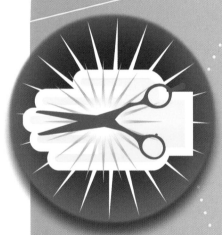

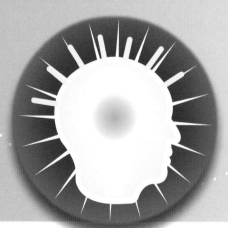

Dexterity
Coordinating the manual skills of holding the scissors, body position and hand position must be mastered as the foundation of cutting perfection.

Discipline
A disciplined approach to haircutting is the key to success.
- Never rush the cut.
- Only cut as much hair as you can control.
- Continually "Read the Hair" as you are cutting.
- Always check your work.

The Parallels

According to **C.C.C. Theory**, there are three parallels that must occur simultaneously for precision cutting:

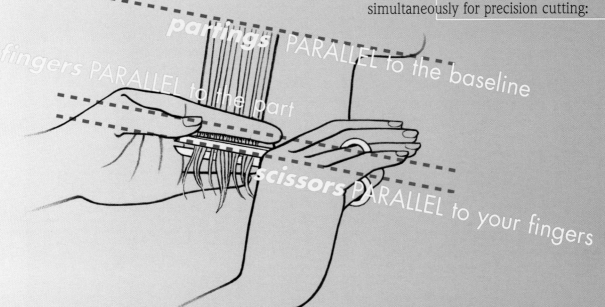

partings PARALLEL to the baseline

fingers PARALLEL to the part

scissors PARALLEL to your fingers

Cutting Perfection

Mastery of **The Law**, **The Skill** and **The Parallels** combined creates the foundation for **Cutting Perfection**.

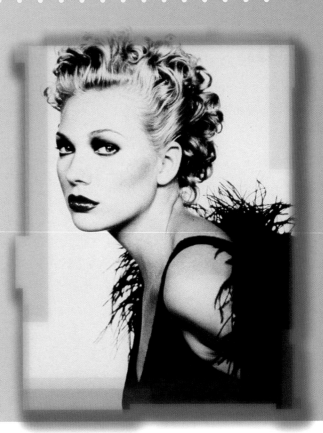

= PERFECTION
(per fek shun), n. an unsurpassable degree of accuracy or excellence.

Textures ...

You will find many different textures of hair on the clients you service. Texture can be produced naturally, chemically or by cutting techniques. Understanding the properties of the various textures will help you predict how the hair reacts to many different cutting techniques.

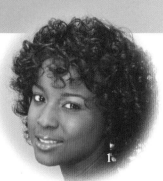

NATURAL TEXTURE

CHEMICAL TEXTURE

CUTTING TEXTURE

Natural Textures

Different lengths of hair are created automatically as a result of daily hair loss and re-growth of hair, which gives a natural variety of edges. Other natural texture influences include growth patterns and shapes of the hair. These factors influence the amount of tension/pressure applied while cutting, the desired length of the haircut and the degrees used for the haircut.

1

rose petals

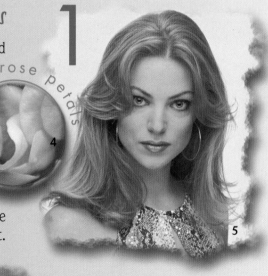

Chemical Textures

2

Chemical textures are created by haircolor, perms, relaxers and/or liquid styling tools such as pomades, oils, gels, glazes, mousses, waxes, etc. Chemicals can add body, shine and dimension to the hair, which produces texture within the overall hair design.

roots

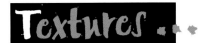

Textures ...

3 Cutting Textures

By cutting hair into various elevations, weight, movement and texture are added to the design. Or, texture is created by using various tools and techniques to create light, airy designs. Cutting textures are divided into three categories:

feathers

1

Constructed Texture: produced by cutting the hair in a compact 0 degree elevation, creating one-length hair. The ends are heavy; therefore producing minimal action in the hair design.

satin

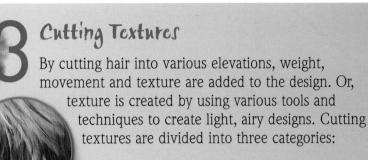

2

Disrupted Texture: a result of cutting the hair with some type of an edge inside the form of the cut, giving action and movement to the hair. Any positive projection haircut will automatically create some disruption.

plant

3

Customized Texture: created with various tools, techniques and cutting shapes. This produces a light, airy and channeled effect within the design.

flower

4

Hair Art Textures Project ...

TEXTURE IS AN IMPORTANT ARTISTIC ELEMENT IN THE DESIGN OF A HAIRCUT.

Textural inspiration can be found all around you. Try paging through your favorite magazine, visiting arts and crafts stores, or simply take a walk outdoors to find examples of **textures** that serve as inspirations for the hairstyles on the following two pages. Place the texture samples in the spaces provided.

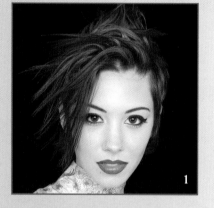

texture sample

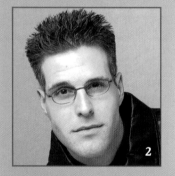

texture sample

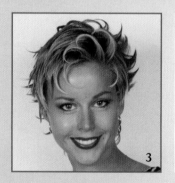

texture sample

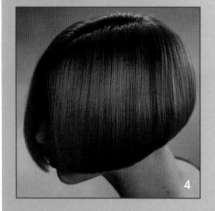

texture sample

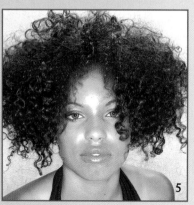

texture sample

texture
sample

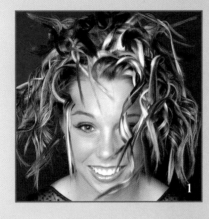

texture
sample

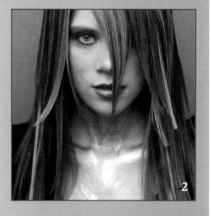

texture
sample

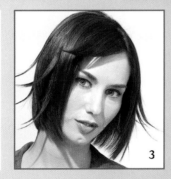

texture
sample

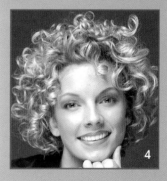

texture
sample

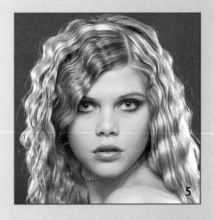

texture
sample

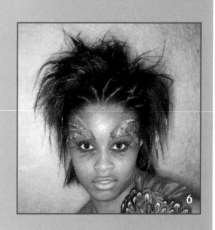

Customizing Textures ...

As your haircutting skills progress beyond the basics, you will want to personalize your cuts by using the various tools and techniques available. Customization of a haircut provides creative expression using movement, separation of textures and versatility of design.

C.C.C.

Theory will help you understand the tools and techniques used to create many different effects. Customization occurs in three areas: the scalp area, the center area and the ends. Each location creates different effects on the hair strand within the overall cut.

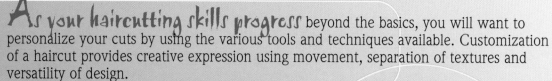

1 Scalp Area Customizing

Occurs anywhere from 1" (2.54 cm) to 2" (5.1 cm) from the scalp, creating a support foundation for volumizing longer hair.

Great textures are enhanced by great products. Sell each client a combination of professional products that will work together to help create the desired results.

2 Center Area Customizing

Occurs in the middle of the strand. Excess hair is reduced, which causes hair to lay closer to the scalp with less volume.

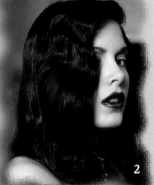

3 End Area Customizing

Is the most popular customization technique. The customizing can occur anywhere on the ends, from the tip up to 3" (7.6 cm) within the ends. Various techniques and tools are used to create a channeled, airy, wispy, or shattered edge effect.

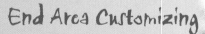

Notch Cutting

Notching can be used as a cutting technique or an end customizing technique. The purpose of notch cutting is to reduce the weight on the ends and blend layers. It is created by cutting serrated points into one inch of the ends of the hair.

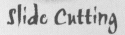

Technique:

1 Stretch the hair flat by holding the hair between your fingers or flat against the scalp.

2 With the tips of the scissors facing inward, cut small diagonal lines in both directions, creating a "V" shape.

1

2

Slide Cutting

is also referred to as slithering or effilating, is an alternate thinning/texturizing technique. It is cutting the hair to graduated lengths using a sliding movement. Sliding uses the shears to blend short to long strands within a small area.

Technique:

1 Release a small section of hair and hold it between your fingers with tension.

2 In an open position, glide the scissors through the hair that is fed into the blades in an angle or arc formation.

3 It is best to work in front of the client when slide cutting on the right side and stand behind the client when slide cutting the left side. (Or, work on the opposite sides when cutting left-handed.)

3

Slicing / Backcutting

Slicing/backcutting is a miniature sliding technique starting 2" (5.1 cm) from the ends, which creates short to longer strands of hair that appear wispy and separated in texture. This technique removes bulk and adds movement within the length of the haircut.

Technique:

1 With the tips of the scissors in a semi-open position, channel the hair outward to the ends.

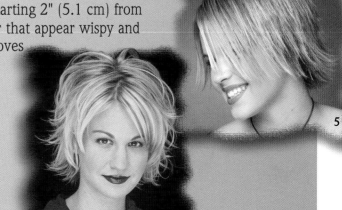

5

4

Point Cutting

Point cutting uses various angles of the scissors to create multiple lengths that blend within the hair ends.

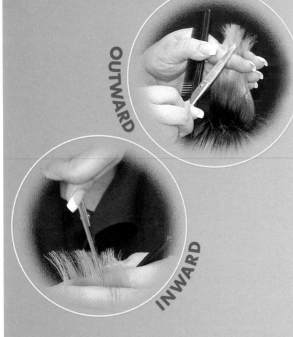

OUTWARD

INWARD

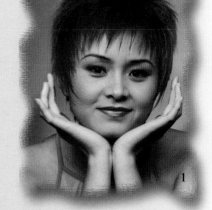

1

Technique:

1. When pointing **outward**, start approximately 3" (7.6 cm) from the hair ends and, with the tips of the scissors facing outward, drag to the ends of the hair.

2. Hold the scissors at an **inward** angle toward the ends of the hair. When pointing inward, lift the hair from the scalp, point the tips of the scissors inward, and cut. The straighter the scissors angle, the less hair that is removed.

Disruption Cutting

Disruption cutting is used to create disruptive texture in the volume area of the head.

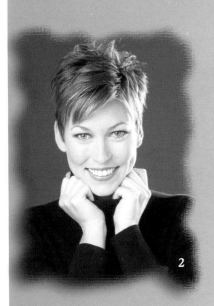

2

Technique:

1. Backcomb a 1" to 2" (2.54 cm to 5.1 cm) square section of the hair (depending upon density) firmly toward the scalp.

2. Cut with the scissors pointing into the ends from the interior of the strand toward the outer edge of the hair.

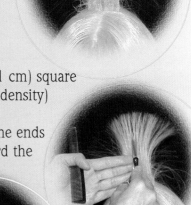

Weave Cutting

Weave cutting scissors (also known as notching, channeling, alpha and more) are used to create special effects into the hair strands. The spacing of the scissors teeth/notches, the depth of the teeth/notches, and the angle of the blades combine to create the special effects on the hair strands.

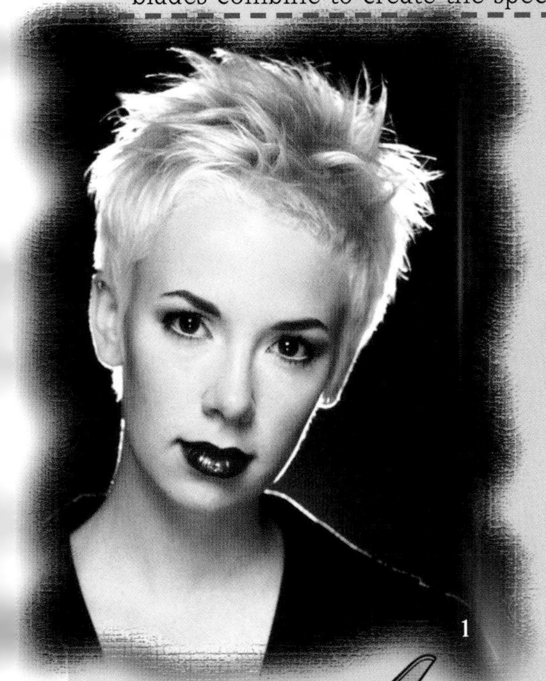

The desired textural special effects can also be created with a standard scissors, using a weave cutting technique. To texturize with a standard scissors, follow these steps:

1 Always work on damp hair.

2 Open the scissors completely, then weave in and out as if weaving haircoloring highlights. Weave thin, medium or heavy strands, depending on the desired effect.

3 Slide the scissors out to 1/3, 1/2 or 2/3 the distance from the root to the ends of the hair, depending on the desired texture and length of hair.

4 Repeat this process as needed on each section of hair, until the desired effect is created.

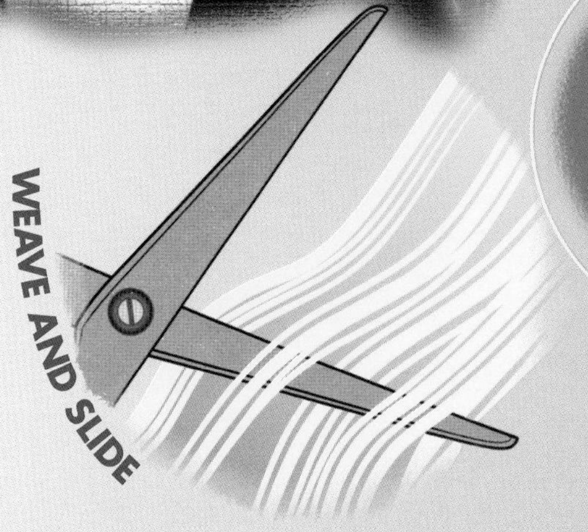

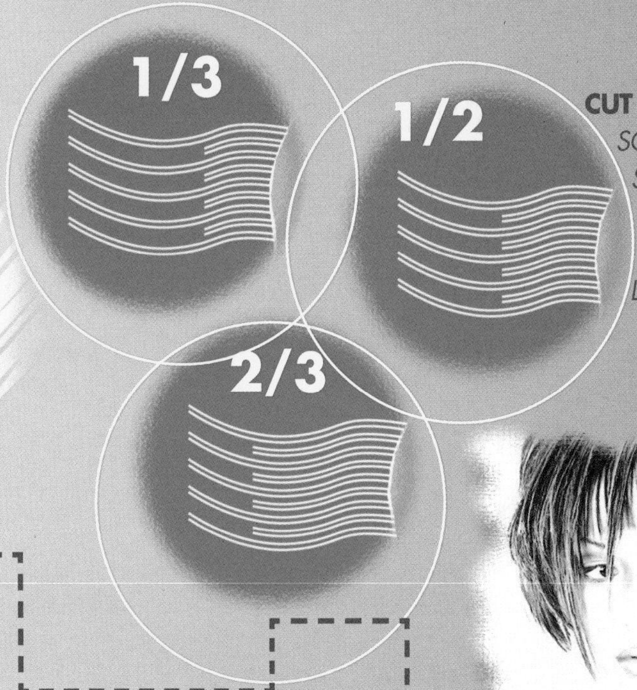

1

WEAVE AND SLIDE

1/3

1/2

2/3

CUT LINE
SOME INTERIOR STRANDS OF THE HAIR ARE SHORTER THAN THE EXTERIOR LENGTHS.

2

"Remember: after weaving the strands to be cut, be sure to cut them at the same angle as the exterior cutting line!"

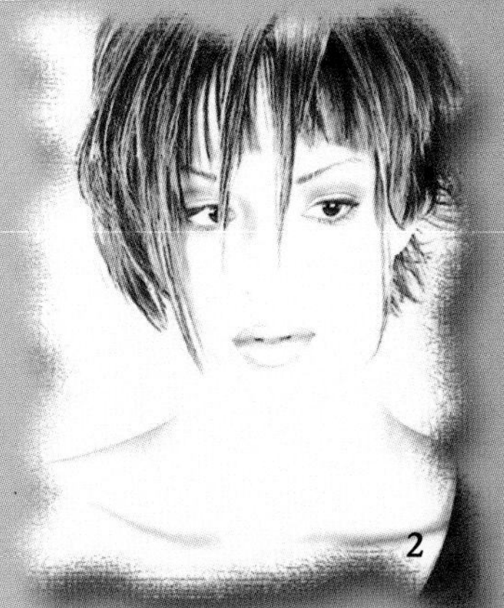

Customizing Textures

Razor Short Stroke

Razor short stroke creates soft and light lines with jagged ends, resulting in a blending of lengths.

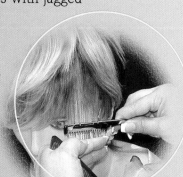

Technique:

1 Position the razor on top of the hair strand, and in an upward and downward motion, cut the ends to produce a line.

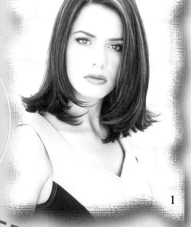

Razor Tapering

Razor tapering is a technique that produces shorter lengths at the base, which support the longer lengths, creating fullness and volume.

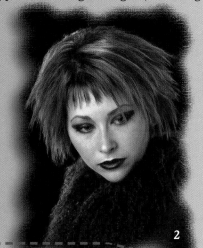

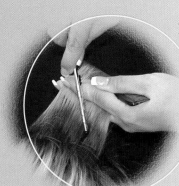

Technique:

1 Using the tip of the razor, cut small intermittent strands of hair approximately 1/2" (1.3 cm) to 1" (2.54 cm) away from the scalp.

Rolling Razor

Razor/comb alternation (also called rolling razor) is used to remove bulk and volume from the hair, allowing the hair to lay closer to the head.

Technique:

1 Rotate the razor and comb on top of the strands of hair.
2 Apply minimum tension to the razor.
3 Determine razor angle for desired effects: the flatter the razor, the less hair that is removed.

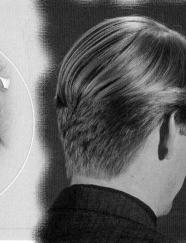

Customizing Textures • Razor Techniques

Side Slicing

Side slicing produces a light, airy blending of lengths, giving movement to the ends.

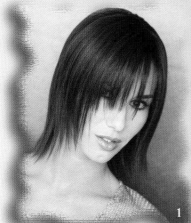

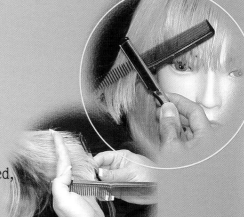

Technique:

1 Hold a large section of hair between the index and middle fingers or with a comb.

2 With the razor held in a vertical position, slide the tip of the razor back and forth across the ends.

3 If only one direction of sliding is used, only one movement is created.

Cuticle Scraping

Cuticle scraping produces a highly texturized effect, moving from the ends to the scalp area.
Caution: Avoid this technique on fine, thin, textured hair.

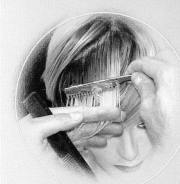

Technique:

1 Hold hair between the fingers and position the razor blade flat on the hair strand.

2 Move the razor down the strand of hair against the grain, scraping the cuticle off.

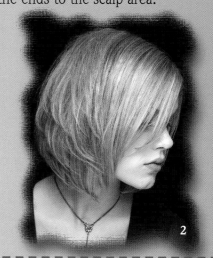

Backcombing

Backcombing with a razor is used to create texture throughout the volume area.

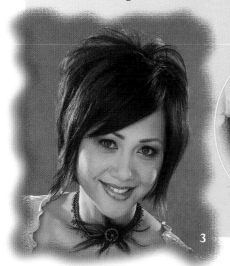

Technique:

1 Begin at the ends, holding the hair between your fingers.

2 Position the razor blade perpendicular to the hair strand, then slide down to the scalp using a backcombing technique. This creates multiple lengths within the ends and center of the strand.

Customizing Textures Project ...

Studying architectural structures and buildings helps you to understand the concepts of form, design and texture. Likewise, studying hairstyles helps you to understand those same concepts.

Examine the gallery of haircuts shown below and identify which texturizing technique may have been used to create each finished cut. Remember, many texturizing techniques are used to create similar effects. Therefore, choose the technique that is the closest match to the finished haircut design.

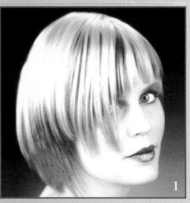

1

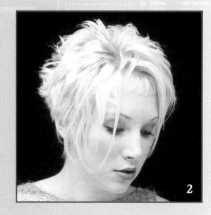

2

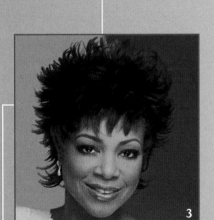

3

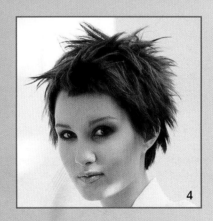

4

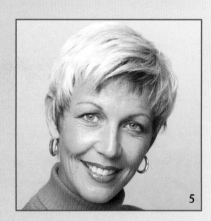

5

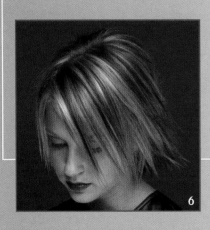

6

CUSTOMIZING TEXTURE TECHNIQUES

1 SLICING/BACKCUTTING   **4** RAZOR TAPERING

2 DISRUPTION CUTTING   **5** SIDE SLICING

3 POINT CUTTING   **6** RAZOR SHORT STROKE

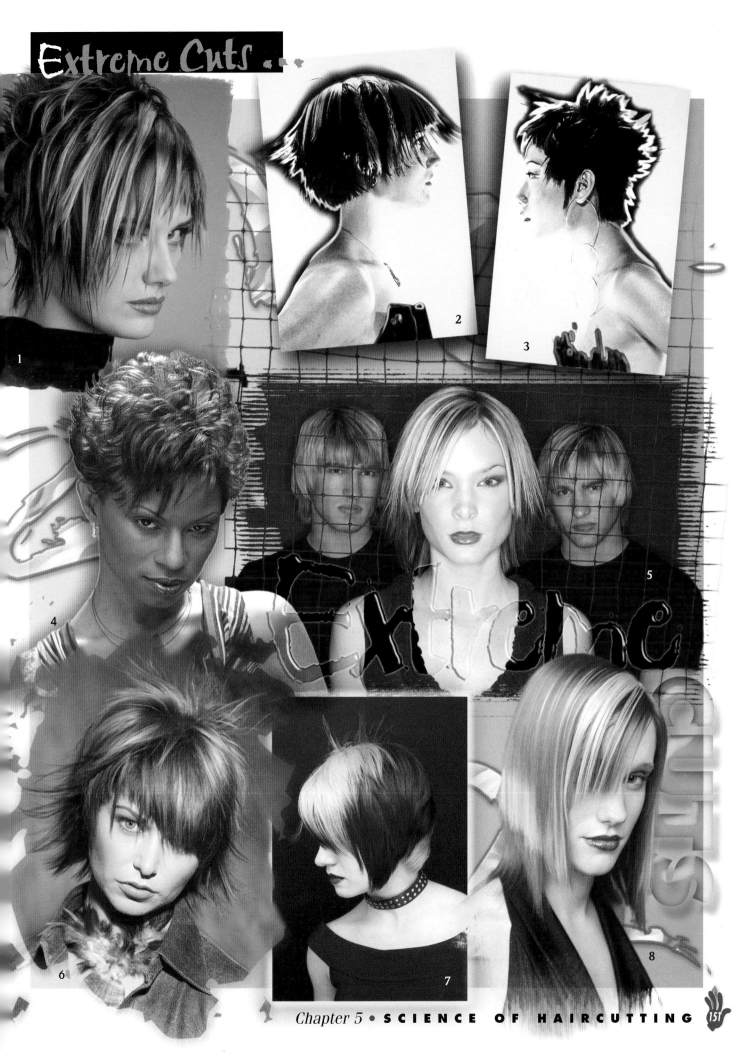

Extreme Cuts

1

2

3

4

5

6

7

8

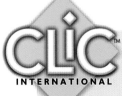

Science of Haircutting REVIEW QUESTIONS

MATCHING

_____ 1. Can be created with a scissors or razor.   **A.** Hypothesis

_____ 2. A technique used to remove bulk from the hair.   **B.** Weave cutting

_____ 3. The straight area between two points on a curved surface.   **C.** The Scientific Method

_____ 4. Can be produced naturally, chemically or by cutting techniques.   **D.** LAW

_____ 5. A tentative assumption about what is causing a future event.   **E.** Customized textures

_____ 6. Produced by cutting the hair at 0 degrees.   **F.** Rolling razor

_____ 7. Can be performed with traditional or weave-cut scissors.   **G.** Constructed texture

_____ 8. 360 degrees   **H.** Texture

_____ 9. Used to develop theories and predict future results.   **I.** Cutting plane

_____ 10. The confidence to cut any length, angles and weight of hair.   **J.** Degrees in a circle

TRUE OR FALSE

_____ 1. Sliding uses the scissors to blend short to long strands within a small section of hair.

_____ 2. The cutting planes can be identified as the area between the two points where the comb leaves the head.

_____ 3. Always cut as much hair at one time as possible to save time between clients.

_____ 4. According to "The Parallels," the partings should always be parallel to the baseline, the fingers should be parallel to the partings, and the scissors should be parallel to your fingers.

_____ 5. Customized textures are the result of growth patterns and shapes of the hair.

_____ 6. Chemical textures are created by haircolor, perms, relaxers and/or liquid styling tools.

_____ 7. Disrupted texture is automatically created within negative elevation haircuts.

_____ 8. Customizing can only occur in the ends of the hair strand.

_____ 9. Notch cutting is created by cutting serrated points into one inch of the ends of the hair.

_____ 10. A circle is actually a series of tangent lines connected at the 360 degree points.

STUDENT'S NAME   DATE   GRADE

HAIRCUTTING

Part of the Webster's dictionary definition of the word perfection is "an unsurpassable degree of accuracy or excellence." My own personal passion for perfection began as a young boy, competing in various school contests. In high school sports and gymnastics competitions, that passion continued. Later, when I entered the field of professional cosmetology the passion remained strong, and it still motivates me to this day.

perfection (per fek shun), n. an unsurpassable degree of accuracy or excellence.

My passion for perfection has led to many professional accomplishments for me. As a young stylist just new to the profession, I entered and won many regional, national and international hair competitions. As a salon owner, I identified a lack of proper mentoring and development of new stylists, and therefore opened my own beauty school. And today, as a veteran of the cosmetology industry, I have identified some weaknesses within the educational and testing systems, and therefore created the CLiC system you are using now!

In this book, I share a lifetime of knowledge of internationally acclaimed haircutting methods and techniques. Mastering these techniques is a great beginning for your own personal passion for perfection. I have always said, "A haircut is only good when it's GREAT!" In order to give great haircuts, you must master and perfect the arts of our trade. Once you learn about the professional haircutting tools and their proper use, your next task is to PRACTICE using the tools until you have developed the precision and speed necessary to work in the salon. Dedication is key to developing your professional skills.

As you study cosmetology, think about your own personal passions and goals. Do you want to be known as the best stylist in your salon ... in your city ... in your state ... in the world?? Remember, if you are passionate about your craft you will be successful. With passion and conviction, there is no limit to what you can accomplish.

Our industry offers a world of opportunities and rewards to those with a passion for their craft. I challenge you to challenge yourself, and be the very best that you can be. Success is out there waiting for you with open arms!

Go for it!

Randy Rick

savàge

audace

boxed bob

sliding wedge

asymmetrical

windblown bob

fru fru

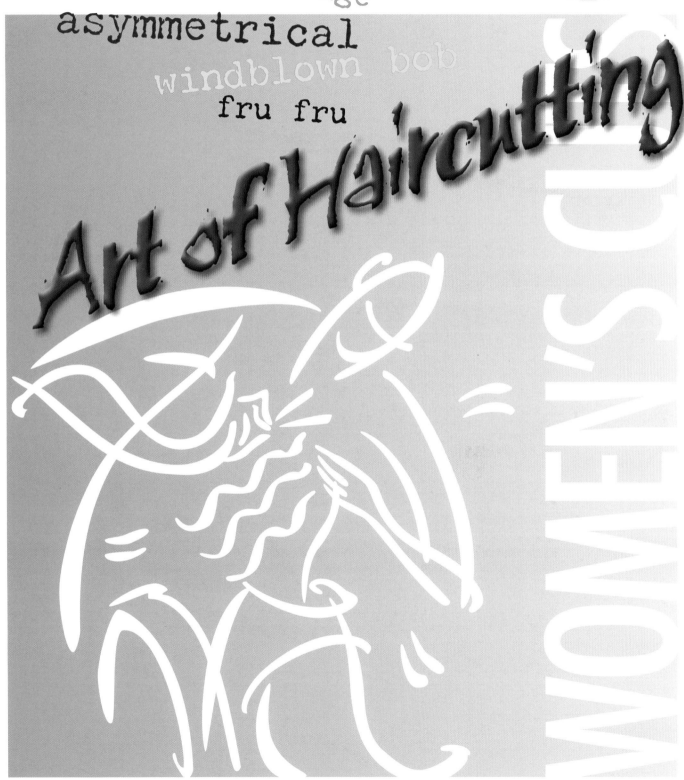

Art of Haircutting

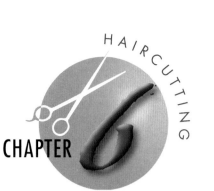

HAIRCUTTING

CHAPTER 6

WOMEN'S DESIGNS

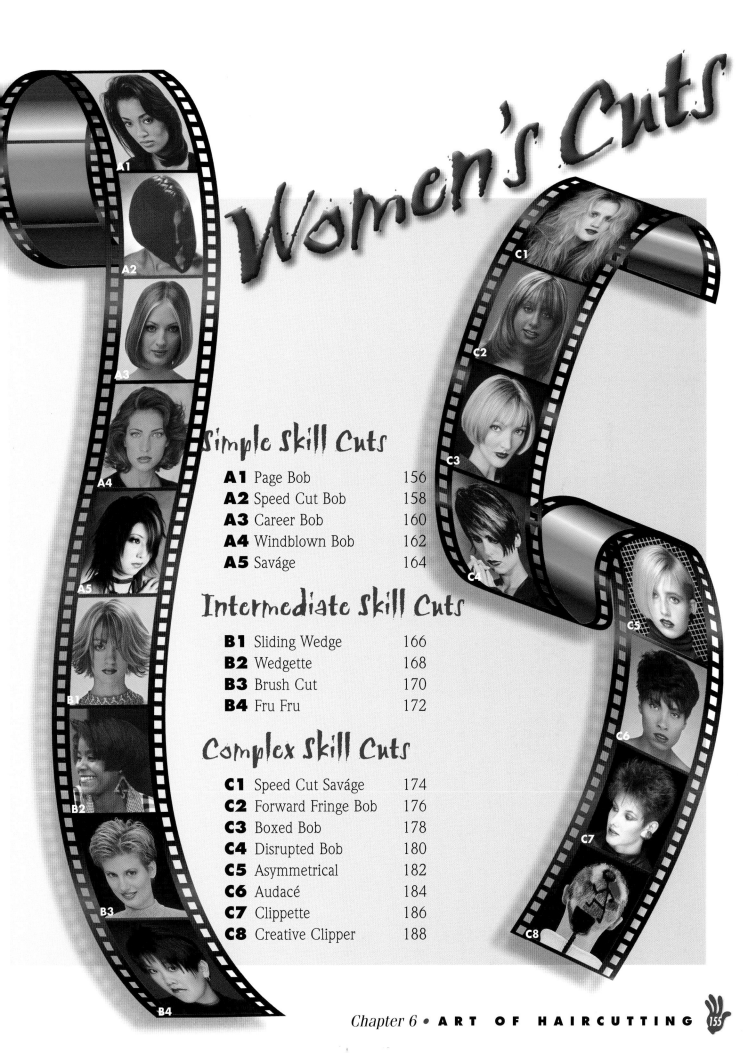

Women's Cuts

Simple Skill Cuts

Intermediate Skill Cuts

Complex Skill Cuts

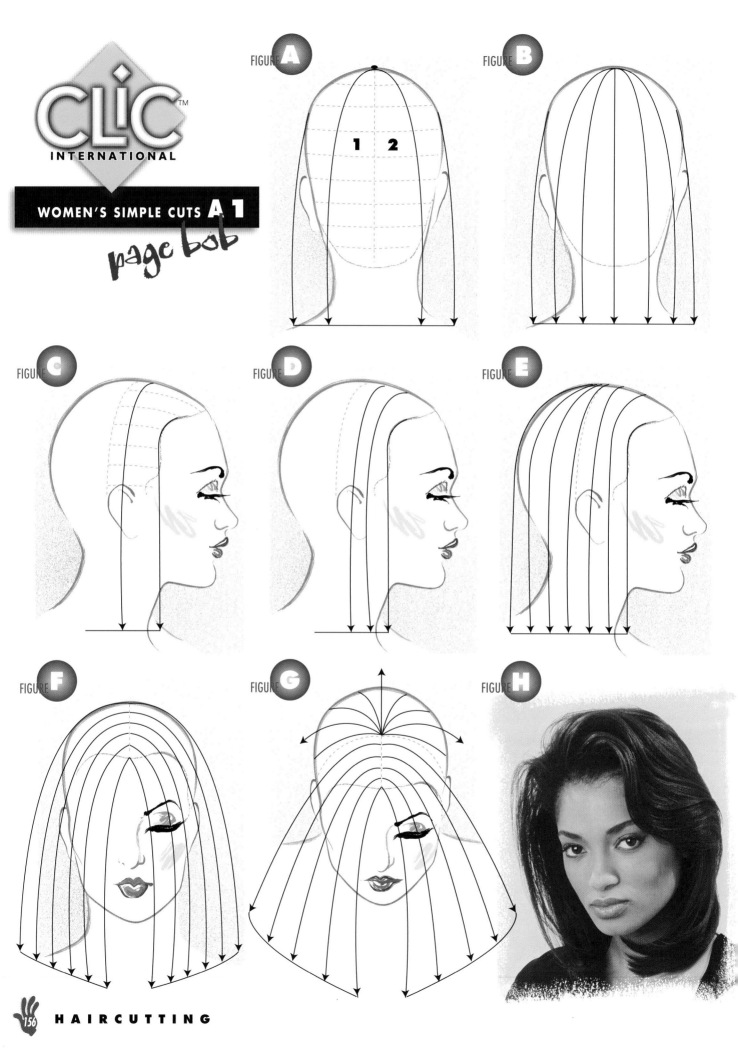

CLiC™
INTERNATIONAL

WOMEN'S SIMPLE CUTS **A1**

page bob

FIGURE **A**

1 **2**

FIGURE **B**

FIGURE **C**

FIGURE **D**

FIGURE **E**

FIGURE **F**

FIGURE **G**

FIGURE **H**

HAIRCUTTING

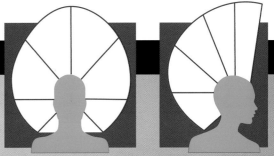

A1 page bob

OBJECTIVE

Master the PAGE BOB, a classic, shoulder-length style. Cut at 0 degrees elevation with minimum tension, the PAGE BOB is a negative, one-length cut. The head is divided into four (4) quarters. A horizontal baseline is cut.

TOOLS & MATERIALS

- Neck Strip
- Towels (2)
- Cape
- All-Purpose Brush
- Shampoo
- Shampoo Comb
- Conditioner
- Cutting Comb
- Clips or Clamps
- Standard 5" (12.7 cm) Scissors
- Liquid Styling Product
- Airformer
- Brushes
- Finishing Spray
- Client Record Card/File

PROCEDURE

"The Client Consultation is an important part of your professional service. Be sure to complete this step prior to each client service you provide. Your successful retail sales and customer satisfaction rates depend upon it!"

1. Drape the client in preparation for the service.
2. Thoroughly brush the client's hair to remove knots, tangles and hairspray.
3. Cleanse the hair with shampoo. Rinse thoroughly and shampoo again. Rinse.
4. Apply the appropriate conditioning product for the client's needs. Rinse thoroughly and towel dry.
5. Comb the hair to remove tangles.
6. Section the hair for the PAGE BOB and secure it with clips/clamps.
7. Perform the haircut as follows:

   A. Divide the back of the head from the control axis into two (2) sections. Part the hair using horizontal lines. Bring all hair down to the baseline and cut at 0 degrees elevation.

   B. Crosscheck the hair using vertical planes.

   C. Part the front 1/3 (0.84cm) of the head using horizontal lines. Bring hair down to the baseline and cut at a 0 degrees elevation, blending with the horizontal line from the back baseline.

   D. Check the hair in vertical planes in its natural fall direction. Repeat on opposite side.

   E. Cut hair horizontally at 0 degrees elevation in vertical planes, blending the front and back areas of the head.

   F. When combed forward to the face, the left and right sides come to a point in the front of the head. Do not remove this point, as the hair will become shorter when combed in its natural fall distribution.

   G. Check and blend all areas, allowing the hair to fall naturally.

   H. Finished design.

8. Apply the liquid styling tool of choice to the hair.
9. Airform the hair to create the desired style.
10. Apply finishing spray to hold the completed style.
11. Follow standard clean-up procedures.
12. Document the Client Record/File.

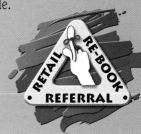

EVALUATION

GRADE

STUDENT'S NAME

ID#

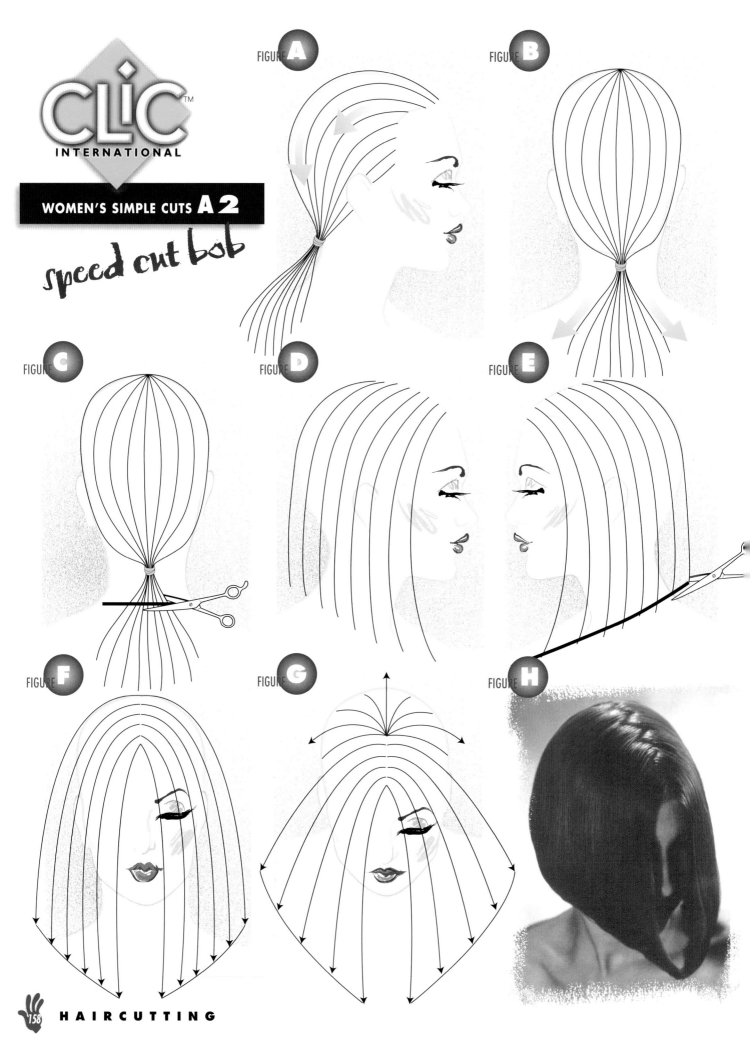

CLiC™
INTERNATIONAL

WOMEN'S SIMPLE CUTS A2

speed cut bob

FIGURE A

FIGURE B

FIGURE C

FIGURE D

FIGURE E

FIGURE F

FIGURE G

FIGURE H

HAIRCUTTING

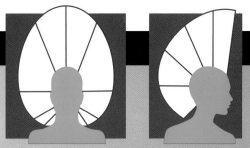

A2 *speed cut bob*

OBJECTIVE

Learn to create a SPEED CUT BOB, a quick and fashionable cut that gives motion and a carefree swing to the hair. A squeeze cutting technique is used to create this low degree haircut. A slight amount of stacking is created by the compacting of hair around the rubber band. The cut begins at the nape area, which creates slightly longer lengths in the front and forms a diagonal forward motion to the face.

TOOLS & MATERIALS

- Neck Strip
- Towels (2)
- Cape
- All-Purpose Brush
- Shampoo
- Shampoo Comb
- Conditioner
- Cutting Comb
- Clips or Clamps
- Standard 5" (12.7 cm) Scissors
- Standard 6" (15.2 cm) Scissors
- Rubber Band
- Liquid Styling Product
- Airformer
- Brushes
- Finishing Spray
- Client Record Card/File

PROCEDURE

"The Client Consultation is an important part of your professional service. Be sure to complete this step prior to each client service you provide. Your successful retail sales and customer satisfaction rates depend upon it!"

1. Drape the client in preparation for the service.
2. Thoroughly brush the client's hair to remove knots, tangles and hairspray.
3. Cleanse the hair with shampoo. Rinse thoroughly and shampoo again. Rinse.
4. Apply the appropriate conditioning product for the client's needs. Rinse thoroughly and towel dry.
5. Comb the hair to remove tangles.
6. Section the hair for the SPEED CUT BOB and secure it with clips/clamps.
7. Perform the haircut as follows:
   A. Comb all hair away from the face. Create tension by holding the hair in the palm of your hand. Tightly position rubber band parallel to the hairline in the center of the nape to create a cutting ponytail.
   B. With the head position straight, comb, squeeze and spread hair evenly into a ponytail.
   C. Determine the length, making sure the hair is combed flat and ribbon smooth for control. With the rubber band in place, position fingers and cut a horizontal line at 0 degrees.

   D. After the hair is cut, release the rubber band and you will see a diagonal forward motion from short in the back to longer in the front. The ends will appear uneven, but the foundation of the diagonal should be evident. **Caution: Hold hand over rubber band when removing to prevent a recoil action.**
   E. This is a profile view of the opposite side, short at the nape and longer toward the front. To check the cut, clean up the baseline around the outer perimeter as needed.
   F. Check for well-balanced symmetry throughout the head.
   G. Comb the front hair forward to a point in front of the face. Use this point as a visual guide to connect and balance both sides. The overview from above shows how the hair falls into its natural state.
   H. Finished design.
8. Apply the liquid styling tool of choice to the hair.
9. Airform the hair to create the desired style.
10. Apply finishing spray to hold the completed style.
11. Follow standard clean-up procedures.
12. Document the Client Record/File.

EVALUATION

GRADE

STUDENT'S NAME

ID#

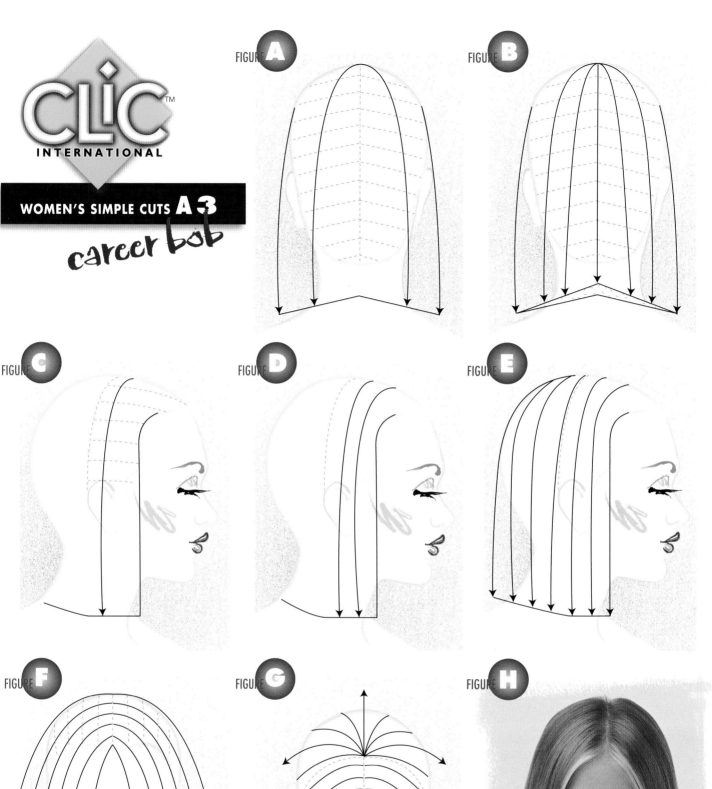

CLiC™
INTERNATIONAL

WOMEN'S SIMPLE CUTS A3

career bob

FIGURE **A**

FIGURE **B**

FIGURE **C**

FIGURE **D**

FIGURE **E**

FIGURE **F**

FIGURE **G**

FIGURE **H**

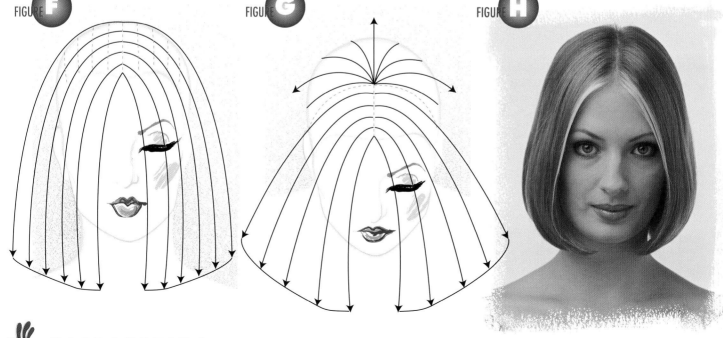

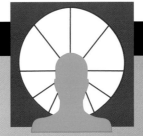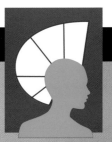

OBJECTIVE

Create the classic, well-balanced, low maintenance CAREER BOB, a low graduated cut. A slight amount of stacking is created by the tension used in cutting. An inverted "V" baseline is cut in the back. Begin the cut at the back and create slightly longer lengths in the front 1/3 (0.84cm) of the head by cutting a diagonal baseline.

TOOLS & MATERIALS

- Neck Strip
- Towels (2)
- Cape
- All-Purpose Brush
- Shampoo
- Shampoo Comb
- Conditioner
- Cutting Comb
- Clips or Clamps
- Standard 5" (12.7 cm) Scissors
- Liquid Styling Product
- Airformer
- Brushes
- Finishing Spray
- Client Record Card/File

PROCEDURE

"The Client Consultation is an important part of your professional service. Be sure to complete this step prior to each client service you provide. Your successful retail sales and customer satisfaction rates depend upon it!"

1. Drape the client in preparation for the service.
2. Thoroughly brush the client's hair to remove knots, tangles and hairspray.
3. Cleanse the hair with shampoo. Rinse thoroughly and shampoo again. Rinse.
4. Apply the appropriate conditioning product for the client's needs. Rinse thoroughly and towel dry.
5. Comb the hair to remove tangles.
6. Section the hair for the CAREER BOB and secure it with clips/clamps.
7. Perform the haircut as follows:

   A. From the control axis, divide the back of the head into two (2) main sections, left and right. Make diagonal partings, that gradually become more horizontal to conform to the curve of the head. Cut in a slight diagonal forward motion with maximum tension at the indentation zone.

   B. Distribute the hair using vertical planes.

   C. The front view shows the front 1/3 (0.84cm) of the head is cut horizontally to blend with the back. Carry the partings throughout the front 1/3 (0.84cm) section. Use minimal tension when cutting over the ears and

   hairline areas to create a mild positive elevation.

   D. Distribute the hair to the established guide. Cut and clean the baseline. Repeat on the opposite side.

   E. After all the hair is cut and in its natural distribution, re-blend the back and front lengths.

   F. Comb hair forward to a point in the front of the face (points create weight). This point must remain to prevent the hair from becoming shorter when it falls in its natural distribution.

   G. Check and blend all areas, allowing the hair to fall in its natural distribution.

   H. Finished design.

8. Apply the liquid styling tool of choice to the hair.
9. Airform the hair to create the desired style.
10. Apply finishing spray to hold the completed style.
11. Follow standard clean-up procedures.
12. Document the Client Record/File.

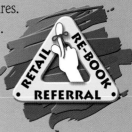

EVALUATION

GRADE

STUDENT'S NAME

ID#

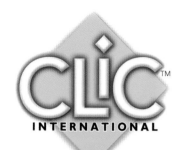

WOMEN'S SIMPLE CUTS A4

windblown bob

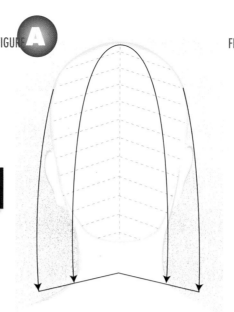

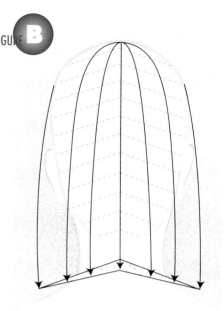

FIGURE C
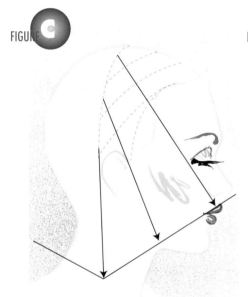

FIGURE D
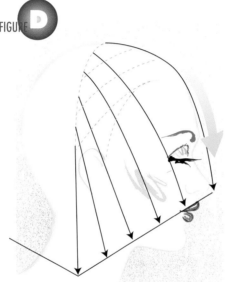

FIGURE E
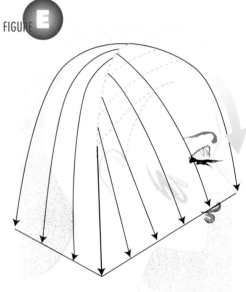

FIGURE F
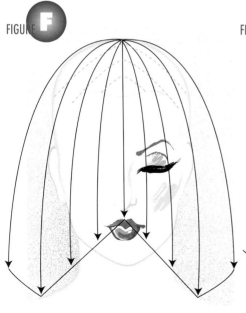

FIGURE G
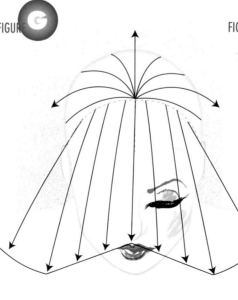

FIGURE H
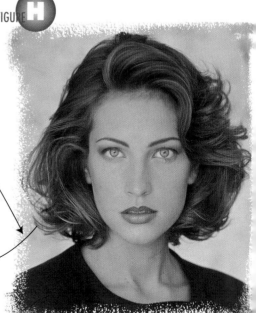

A4 *windblown bob*

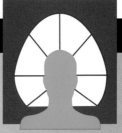
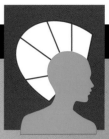

OBJECTIVE

Learn the WINDBLOWN BOB, a cut combining the fullness and volume of a classic bob in the back with textured softness framing the face in an unconstructed design. The back is a positive low elevation cut. Positive elevation is created in the front 1/3 (0.84cm) of the head by shifting the hair forward to an established baseline.

TOOLS & MATERIALS

- Neck Strip
- Towels (2)
- Cape
- All-Purpose Brush
- Shampoo
- Shampoo Comb
- Conditioner
- Cutting Comb
- Clips or Clamps
- Standard 5" (12.7 cm) Scissors
- Texturizing Tool of Choice
- Liquid Styling Product
- Airformer
- Brushes
- Finishing Spray
- Client Record Card/File

PROCEDURE

"The Client Consultation is an important part of your professional service. Be sure to complete this step prior to each client service you provide. Your successful retail sales and customer satisfaction rates depend upon it!"

1. Drape the client in preparation for the service.
2. Thoroughly brush the client's hair to remove knots, tangles and hairspray.
3. Cleanse the hair with shampoo. Rinse thoroughly and shampoo again. Rinse.
4. Apply the appropriate conditioning product for the client's needs. Rinse thoroughly and towel dry.
5. Comb the hair to remove tangles.
6. Section the hair for the WINDBLOWN BOB and secure it with clips/clamps.
7. Perform the haircut as follows:
   A. The baseline in the back of the head is cut in an inverted "V". Create diagonal partings that become more horizontal and conform to the curve of the head while moving up the head.
   B. Cut the hair with tension to create a slight stacking effect. All hair must be distributed in vertical planes and cut horizontally.
   C. The baseline in the front 1/3 (0.84cm) is a diagonal line from the lip (mouth) to the established length at the back of the ear. Part around the hairline, almost vertically, then change to diagonal back.
   D. Cut the hair to the established guide using a shifting technique. Continue shifting at the top of the head to create more layering. Repeat on the opposite side.
   E. The hair in the back 2/3 (1.7cm) is cut in its natural distribution and the hair in the front 1/3 (0.84cm) is shifted forward. The hair above the ear is shifted less to blend with the back lengths.
   F. Shift hair forward in the front and blend with the lengths in the back. Use less shifting above the ear area.
   G. Blend and check all lengths in their natural distribution.
   H. Finished design.
8. Apply the liquid styling tool of choice to the hair.
9. Airform the hair to create the desired style.
10. Apply finishing spray to hold the completed style.
11. Follow standard clean-up procedures.
12. Document the Client Record/File.

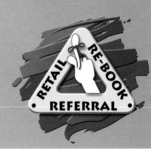

EVALUATION

GRADE

STUDENT'S NAME

ID#

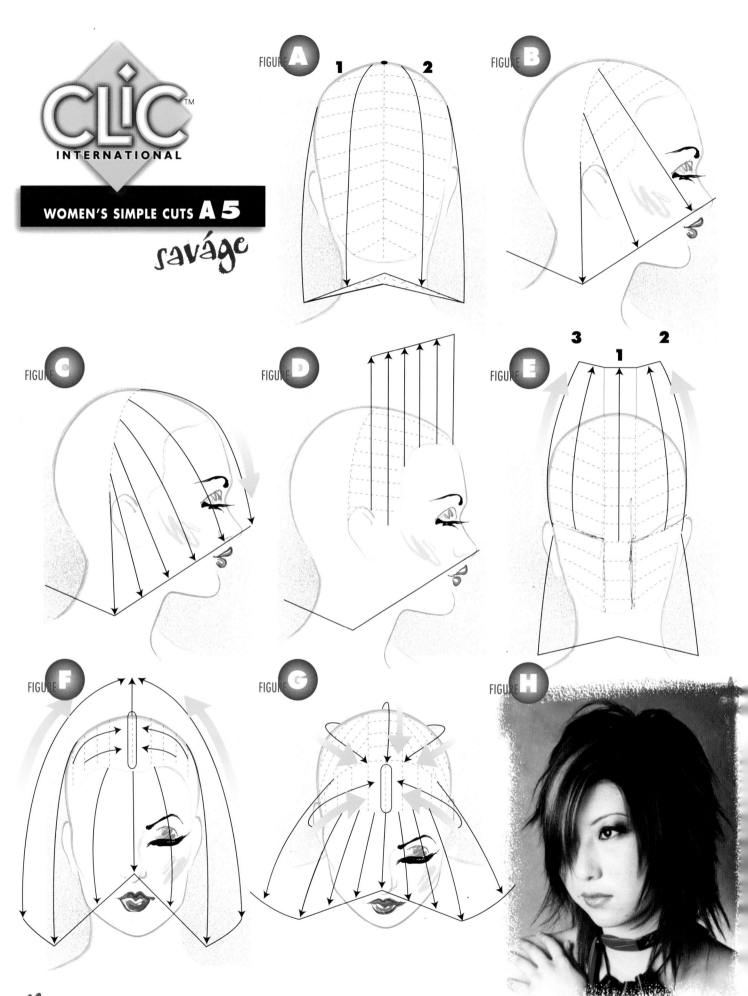

WOMEN'S SIMPLE CUTS A 5

saváge

FIGURE A

FIGURE B

FIGURE C

FIGURE D

FIGURE E

FIGURE F

FIGURE G

FIGURE H

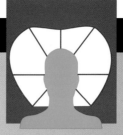
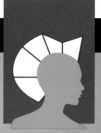

A5 savage

OBJECTIVE

Master the SAVÁGE, a mid-length cut with stylish shag in an unconstructed design. It is a reverse positive elevation cut. The entire perimeter is cut taking 1/4" (0.6 cm) off the existing baseline. Interior layers are created using a squeeze technique.

TOOLS & MATERIALS

- Neck Strip
- Towels (2)
- Cape
- All-Purpose Brush
- Shampoo
- Shampoo Comb
- Conditioner
- Cutting Comb
- Clips or Clamps
- Standard 5" (12.7 cm) Scissors or Razor
- Texturizing Tool of Choice
- Liquid Styling Product
- Airformer
- Brushes
- Finishing Spray
- Client Record Card/File

PROCEDURE

"The Client Consultation is an important part of your professional service. Be sure to complete this step prior to each client service you provide. Your successful retail sales and customer satisfaction rates depend upon it!"

1. Drape the client in preparation for the service.
2. Thoroughly brush the client's hair to remove knots, tangles and hairspray.
3. Cleanse the hair with shampoo. Rinse thoroughly and shampoo again. Rinse.
4. Apply the appropriate conditioning product for the client's needs. Rinse thoroughly and towel dry.
5. Comb the hair to remove tangles.
6. Section the hair for the SAVÁGE and secure it with clips.
7. Perform the haircut as follows:

   A. Divide the back of the head into two (2) sections. Use diagonal partings, that gradually become horizontal to conform to the curve of the head. The hair must be cut in its natural distribution using tension to create a low degree, stacking effect.

   B. Begin a diagonal back baseline from the nose to blend with the length established in the back. Use diagonal partings when cutting.

   C. Shift the hair in the front 1/3 (0.84cm) to the baseline to create layering and length increase. Shifting and elevation are used to create more layering. A low elevation is used above the ear to blend with the back lengths. Repeat on opposite side.

   D. Create reverse positive elevation by establishing a 6" (15.2 cm) guide on the top of the head. Cut the top guide anti-head, getting slightly longer toward the face. Create squeeze layering by bringing all hair up and cutting to this guide, using horizontal partings. Repeat on opposite side.

   E. Divide the back of the head into three (3) panels. Cut the center panel first using a small section of previously cut hair on the top of the head as a guide. Bring all hair up and use a squeezing technique. Cut the side back panels in the same manner, blending the layering in the front of the head and the center back panel.

   F. Check and blend all lengths and layering in the front of the head.

   G. After checking and blending all lengths and layering in the back of the head, check and blend from front to back.

   H. Finished design.

8. Apply the liquid styling tool of choice to the hair.
9. Airform the hair to create the desired style.
10. Apply finishing spray to hold the completed style.
11. Follow standard clean-up procedures.
12. Document the Client Record/File.

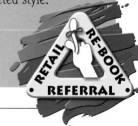

EVALUATION

GRADE

STUDENT'S NAME

ID#

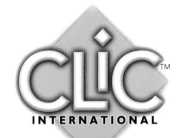

WOMEN'S INTERMEDIATE CUTS B1

sliding wedge

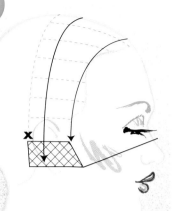

FIGURE A

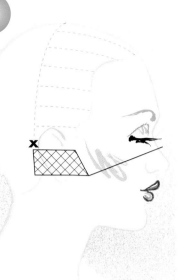

FIGURE B

FIGURE C

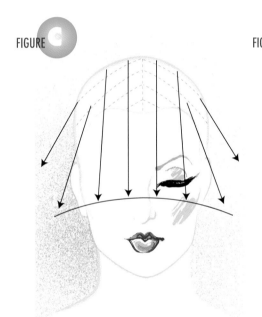

FIGURE D

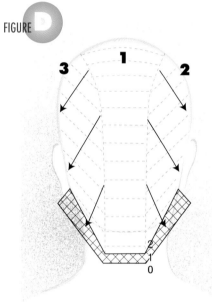

FIGURE E

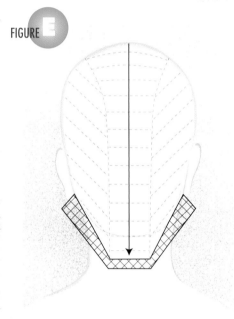

FIGURE F

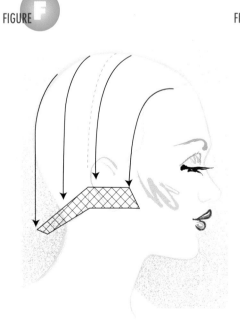

FIGURE G

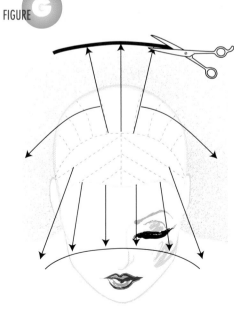

FIGURE H

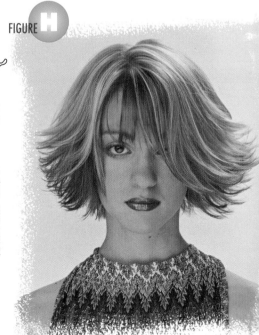

HAIRCUTTING

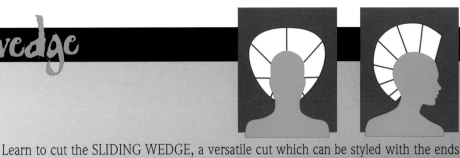
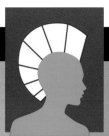

B1 sliding wedge

OBJECTIVE

Learn to cut the SLIDING WEDGE, a versatile cut which can be styled with the ends flipped outward or turned under. This is a classic low positive elevation haircut. A weight line is created where one length hair meets at low elevation. Proper tension and a natural fall distribution are important when performing this cut.

TOOLS & MATERIALS

- Neck Strip
- Towels (2)
- Cape
- All-Purpose Brush
- Shampoo
- Shampoo Comb
- Conditioner
- Cutting Comb
- Clips or Clamps
- Standard 5" (12.7 cm) Scissors
- Razor
- Texturizing Tool of Choice
- Liquid Styling Product
- Airformer
- Brushes
- Finishing Spray
- Client Record Card/File

PROCEDURE

"The Client Consultation is an important part of your professional service. Be sure to complete this step prior to each client service you provide. Your successful retail sales and customer satisfaction rates depend upon it!"

1. Drape the client in preparation for the service.
2. Thoroughly brush the client's hair to remove knots, tangles and hairspray.
3. Cleanse the hair with shampoo. Rinse thoroughly and shampoo again. Rinse.
4. Apply the appropriate conditioning product for the client's needs. Rinse thoroughly and towel dry.
5. Comb the hair to remove tangles.
6. Section the hair for the SLIDING WEDGE and secure it with clips/clamps.
7. Perform the haircut as follows:
   A. Cut the front 1/3 (0.84cm) of the head first. Establish a horizontal baseline just above the ear lobe. Bring all hair to this baseline and cut using one- (1) finger elevation. Make horizontal partings. Cut the hair with tension in its natural fall distribution to create the desired stacking.
   B. This illustrates the stacking created at the ear. The "X" indicates the weight line created by the long hair meeting the elevation.
   C. Create a front baseline from the center of the nose to meet the horizontal baseline on the side. Use diagonal back partings. Shift hair forward, moving from the volume zone down to the side. Blend elevation at the ear. Repeat on opposite side.
   D. Divide the back of the head into three (3) panels

following the curve of the head. Cut the indentation zone first. Establish a horizontal baseline at the nape center plane. Bring all hair down and cut to the baseline using two- (2) finger elevation. Cut the center plane area using natural fall distribution and tension.

   E. Cut the baseline for both sides of the back, blending from the length at the ear to the length established at the center plane nape. Create diagonal partings to conform to the baseline. Cut the hair with tension, using two- (2) finger elevation in its natural fall distribution.
   F. Blend all baselines and elevations by cutting with tension in the natural fall direction.
   G. Shift the hair in the front of the head forward and blend with the stacked horizontal lines created at the ears. Blend hair in its natural fall distribution. At the control zone of the head, hold hair straight up at a 90 degrees elevation and round off the corners. Check and blend haircut.
   H. Finished design.
8. Apply the liquid styling tool of choice to the hair.
9. Airform the hair to create the desired style.
10. Apply finishing spray to hold the completed style.
11. Follow standard clean-up procedures.
12. Document the Client Record/File.

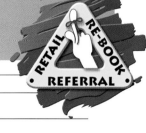

EVALUATION

GRADE

STUDENT'S NAME

ID#

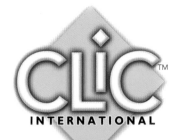

FIGURE **A**

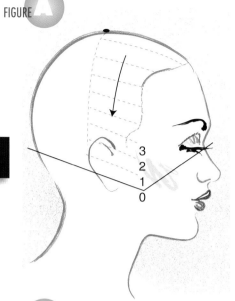

3
2
1
0

FIGURE **B**

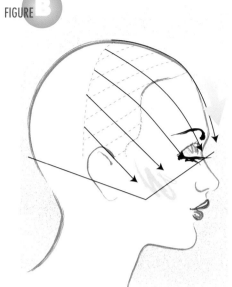

FIGURE **C**

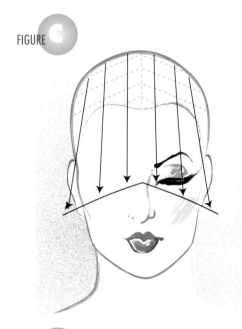

FIGURE **D**

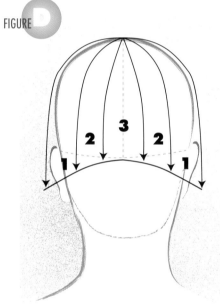

2 3 2
1 1

FIGURE **E**

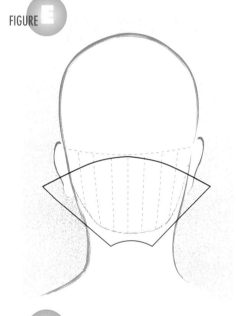

FIGURE **F**

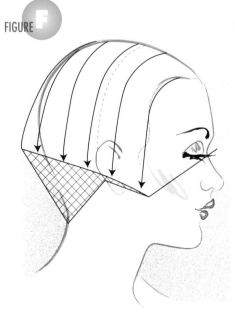

FIGURE **G**

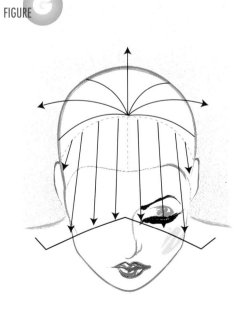

FIGURE **H**

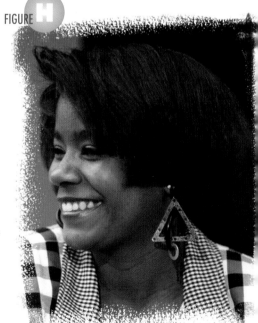

B2 *wedgette*

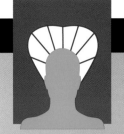
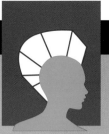

OBJECTIVE

Learn to cut the WEDGETTE, a short, classic look with a tapered back that hugs the neckline. A graduating finger elevation is used to create a soft weight line for this low elevation haircut. Texturizing is utilized to lighten and disrupt the edges.

TOOLS & MATERIALS

- Neck Strip
- Towels (2)
- Cape
- All-Purpose Brush
- Shampoo
- Shampoo Comb
- Conditioner
- Cutting Comb
- Clips or Clamps
- Razor
- Standard 5" (12.7 cm) Scissors
- Texturizing Tool of Choice
- Liquid Styling Product
- Airformer
- Brushes
- Finishing Spray
- Client Record Card/File

PROCEDURE

"The Client Consultation is an important part of your professional service. Be sure to complete this step prior to each client service you provide. Your successful retail sales and customer satisfaction rates depend upon it!"

1. Drape the client in preparation for the service.
2. Thoroughly brush the client's hair to remove knots, tangles and hairspray.
3. Cleanse the hair with shampoo. Rinse thoroughly and shampoo again. Rinse.
4. Apply the appropriate conditioning product for the client's needs. Rinse thoroughly and towel dry.
5. Comb the hair to remove tangles.
6. Section the hair for the WEDGETTE and secure it with clips.
7. Perform the haircut as follows:

   A. Section from the center hairline to the control axis and vertically ear to ear. Subsection the indentation zone (nape) horizontally from top of ear to top of ear. Starting at the front side panel, part a diagonal forward motion line. Cut the baseline guide at 0 degrees. Start by using a one- (1) finger elevation. Continue with the next section using a two- (2) finger elevation. On the third section, you should be at the lower rim zone of the head and using a three- (3) finger elevation. At this point, all hair is brought down and projected out at a three- (3) finger elevation, creating the weight line (X).

   B. Using the bridge of the nose as a reference guide, comb the hair from the frontal bang area forward and cut at 0 degrees (negative elevation). Connect the longest length from the side panel with the frontal bang area and cut on a diagonal back line toward the bridge of the nose.

   C. Comb the hair forward using diagonal back partings. Do not use tension when cutting in the frontal hairline area. A weak hairline will jump up and get too short. Continue to blend the frontal area panels.

   D. In order to create the soft weight line in the back of the head, part horizontally from ear to ear. The guide is cut with a one- (1) finger elevation in the first plane behind the ear. Continue to blend to a two- (2) finger elevation, then to a three- (3) finger elevation at the center plane. Repeat on opposite side.

   E. Cut baseline design into hairline at nape. Graduate from nape to weight line. Take horizontal partings within each plane and cut palm to palm, using a traveling guide up the back of the head. (Optional technique: use vertical sections to connect baseline to weight line.)

   F. Clean and connect the side panels to the baseline using the shortest hair from the side panel and cut to the longest length at the baseline.

   G. Check, clean and personalize the entire structure. Blend all lengths in a natural fall distribution. Texturize to achieve desired special effects.

   H. Finished design.

8. Apply the liquid styling tool of choice to the hair.
9. Airform the hair to create the desired style.
10. Apply finishing spray to hold the completed style.
11. Follow standard clean-up procedures.
12. Document the Client Record/File.

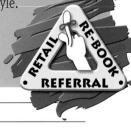

EVALUATION

GRADE

STUDENT'S NAME

ID#

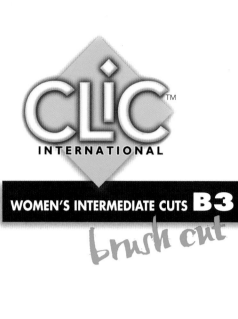

WOMEN'S INTERMEDIATE CUTS **B3**

brush cut

FIGURE **A**

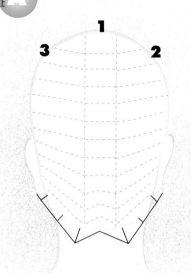

FIGURE **B**

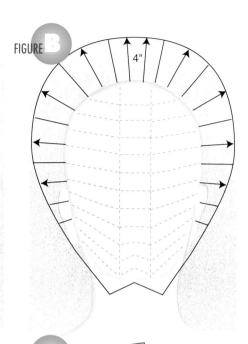

4"

FIGURE **C**

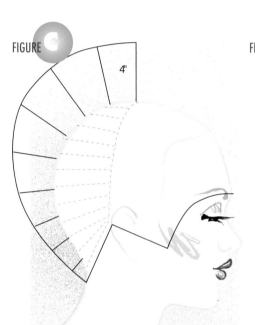

4"

FIGURE **D**

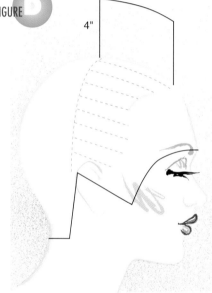

4"

FIGURE **E**

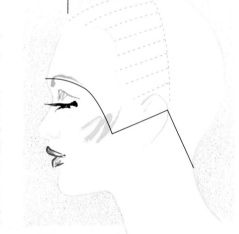

4"

FIGURE **F**

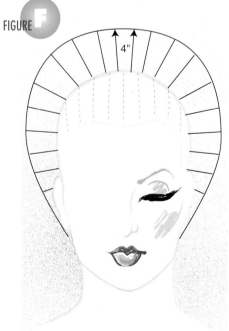

4"

FIGURE **G**

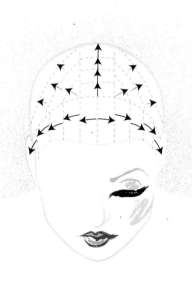

FIGURE **H**

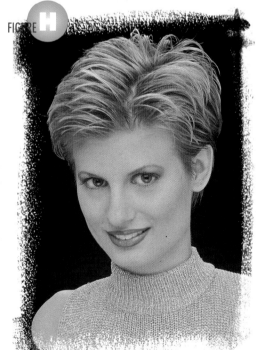

HAIRCUTTING

B3 brush cut

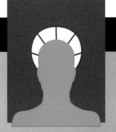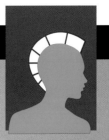

OBJECTIVE

Create the BRUSH CUT, a carefree, sassy style that can be finished loosely with fingers or dried in a smooth, polished look. This layered cut has high elevation in the nape and 90 degrees elevation in the crown. It can be cut using a razor or a combination of scissors and razor.

TOOLS & MATERIALS

- Neck Strip
- Towels (2)
- Cape
- All-Purpose Brush
- Shampoo
- Shampoo Comb
- Conditioner
- Cutting Comb
- Clips or Clamps
- Razor
- Standard 5" (12.7 cm) Scissors
- Texturizing Tool of Choice
- Liquid Styling Product
- Airformer
- Brushes
- Finishing Spray
- Client Record Card/File

PROCEDURE

"The Client Consultation is an important part of your professional service. Be sure to complete this step prior to each client service you provide. Your successful retail sales and customer satisfaction rates depend upon it!"

1. Drape the client in preparation for the service.
2. Thoroughly brush the client's hair to remove knots, tangles and hairspray.
3. Cleanse the hair with shampoo. Rinse thoroughly and shampoo again. Rinse.
4. Apply the appropriate conditioning product for the client's needs. Rinse thoroughly and towel dry.
5. Comb the hair to remove tangles.
6. Section the hair for the BRUSH CUT and secure it with clips/clamps.
7. Perform the haircut as follows:

   A. Divide the back of the head into three (3) panels. Cut an inverted "V" shape in the center plane nape area (#1) at 0 degrees elevation. Moving up the back of the head, graduate to a positive 90 degrees elevation. Cut back side planes (#2 and #3) on a diagonal. Back partings graduate from 0 degrees to 90 degrees.

   B. There is positive 90 degrees elevation in the nape with hair progressing to longer lengths in the crown.

   C. Cut the hair at low elevation above the ear. Then cut the hair using positive elevation to approximately 4" (10.2 cm) in the crown.

   D. Cut a diagonal forward motion baseline at the ear, removing only a slight bit of length. Cut the front baseline by blending from the bridge of the nose to the baseline at the ear. Cut the layering using diagonal partings and reverse high elevation to blend the lengths from the back to the front baseline. Remember to leave some weight at the front hairline.

   E. Repeat the same cutting technique on the other side. Texturize the outer perimeter to create the desired effect.

   F. Check and blend all layering vertically.

   G. Check and blend all areas of the head in its natural fall distribution.

   H. Finished design.

8. Apply the liquid styling tool of choice to the hair.
9. Airform the hair to create the desired style.
10. Apply finishing spray to hold the completed style.
11. Follow standard clean-up procedures.
12. Document the Client Record/File.

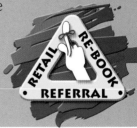

EVALUATION

GRADE

STUDENT'S NAME

ID#

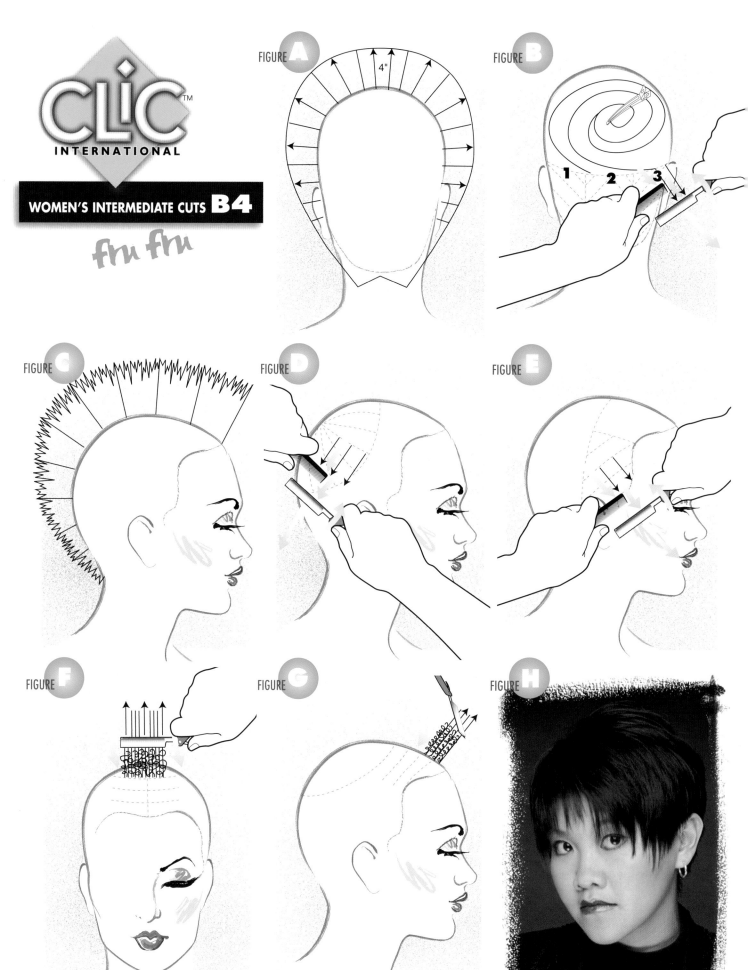

CLiC™
INTERNATIONAL

WOMEN'S INTERMEDIATE CUTS **B4**

fru fru

FIGURE A

4"

FIGURE B

1   2   3

FIGURE C

FIGURE D

FIGURE E

FIGURE F

FIGURE G

FIGURE H

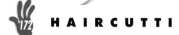

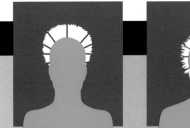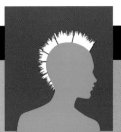

B4 *fru fru*

OBJECTIVE

Design a FRU FRU cut using a series of customizing razor techniques to create soft, wispy edges.

TOOLS & MATERIALS

- Neck Strip
- Towels (2)
- Cape
- All-Purpose Brush
- Shampoo
- Shampoo Comb
- Conditioner
- Cutting Comb
- Clips or Clamps
- Texturizing Scissors
- Razor
- Liquid Styling Product
- Airformer
- Brushes
- Finishing Spray
- Client Record Card/File

PROCEDURE

"The Client Consultation is an important part of your professional service. Be sure to complete this step prior to each client service you provide. Your successful retail sales and customer satisfaction rates depend upon it!"

1. Drape the client in preparation for the service.
2. Thoroughly brush the client's hair to remove knots, tangles and hairspray.
3. Cleanse the hair with shampoo. Rinse thoroughly and shampoo again. Rinse.
4. Apply the appropriate conditioning product for the client's needs. Rinse thoroughly and towel dry.
5. Comb the hair to remove tangles.
6. Section the hair for the FRU FRU and secure it with clips/clamps.
7. Perform the haircut as follows:

   A. Create positive elevation of the hair to see the length arrangements on the head.

   B. Section the nape area below the rim zone from ear to ear and then divide the nape into three panels, working from the left to right. Begin by taking small diagonal back motion partings. Place the razor blade and comb on top of the strands of hair and apply minimal tension. The flatter the razor is positioned, the less hair is removed. The comb lifts while the razor rolls close to the surface to remove slight amounts of hair at a time. This is a Rolling Razor technique.

   C. Notice the disrupted texture achieved by the razor. Mobility and softness will give freedom to the design.

   D. Use the same Rolling Razor technique in the crown area.

   E. Separate the front side panel from the back area. Apply the same technique, using diagonal back partings. Note: Use caution around the face when using a razor.

   F. Proceed to the top of the head. Throughout the volume zone perform Razor Backcombing and Cuticle Scraping customizing techniques with the razor.

   G. Separate two panels; start texturizing from front to back. Razor Backcombing is utilized to create texture throughout the volume zone. Begin at the ends. Holding the hair between your fingers, position the blade perpendicular to the strand and slide down to the scalp as if you were backcombing. Cuticle Scraping produces a highly texturized effect, moving from the ends to the scalp area. Hold the hair between your fingers using maximum tension. Use the edge of the razor by positioning the blade edge flat on the hair strand. Move the razor down the strand of hair against the grain, scraping the cuticle off. **Caution: Avoid this technique on fine, thin textured hair and on damaged or bleached hair.**

   H. Finished design.

8. Apply the liquid styling tool of choice to the hair.
9. Airform the hair to create the desired style.
10. Apply finishing spray to hold the completed style.
11. Follow standard clean-up procedures.
12. Document the Client Record/File.

EVALUATION

_____
_____

GRADE

_____

STUDENT'S NAME

ID#

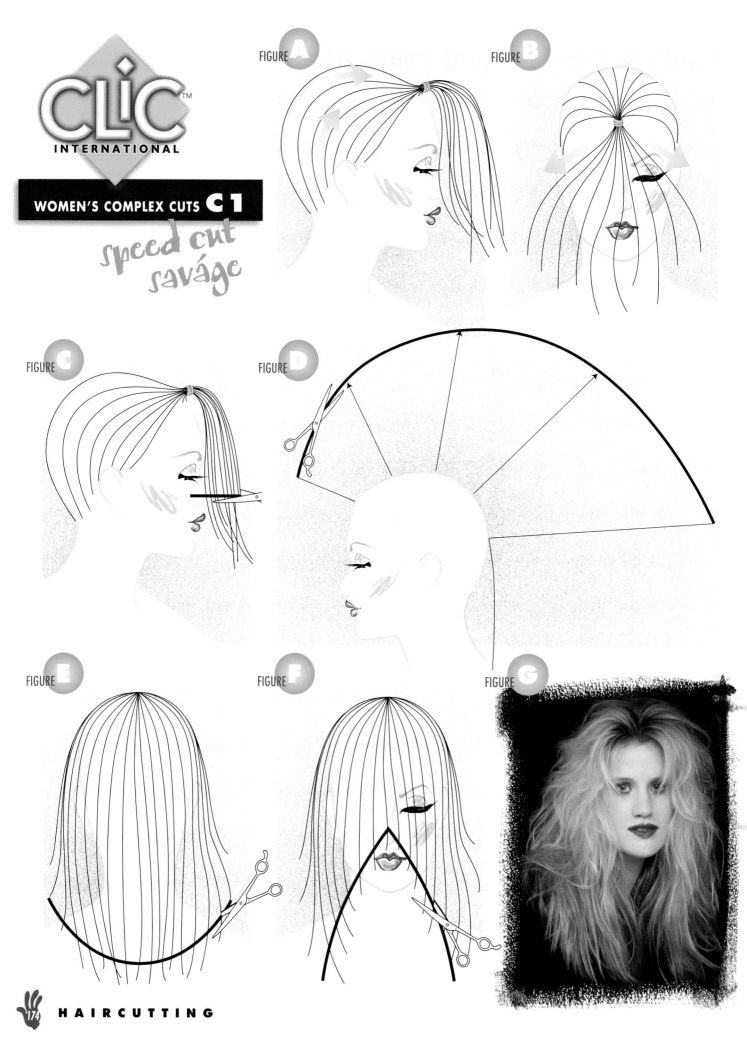

CLiC™
INTERNATIONAL

WOMEN'S COMPLEX CUTS **C 1**

speed cut saváge

FIGURE A

FIGURE B

FIGURE C

FIGURE D

FIGURE E

FIGURE F

FIGURE G

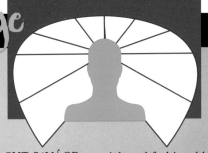
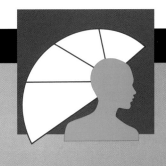

C1 *speed cut saváge*

OBJECTIVE

Learn the SPEED CUT SAVÁGE, a quick and fashionable style combining the versatility of long hair with the fullness of a layered cut. This rubber band cut is performed using the scissors or tool of your choice. The hair is brought to the front hairline and secured with a rubber band prior to cutting.

TOOLS & MATERIALS

- Neck Strip
- Towels (2)
- Cape
- All-Purpose Brush
- Shampoo
- Shampoo Comb
- Conditioner
- Cutting Comb
- Clips or Clamps
- 6" (15.2 cm) Scissors
- Rubber Band
- Razor
- Texturizing Tool of Choice
- Liquid Styling Product
- Airformer
- Brushes
- Finishing Spray
- Client Record Card/File

PROCEDURE

"The Client Consultation is an important part of your professional service. Be sure to complete this step prior to each client service you provide. Your successful retail sales and customer satisfaction rates depend upon it!"

1. Drape the client in preparation for the service.
2. Thoroughly brush the client's hair to remove knots, tangles and hairspray.
3. Cleanse the hair with shampoo. Rinse thoroughly and shampoo again. Rinse.
4. Apply the appropriate conditioning product for the client's needs. Rinse thoroughly and towel dry.
5. Comb the hair to remove tangles.
6. Section the hair for the SPEED CUT SAVÁGE and secure it with clips/clamps.
7. Perform the haircut as follows:

    A. Comb the entire indentation and volume zones to the frontal area. Even distribution is crucial. Be sure to comb all lengths to the frontal area in a smooth, continuous line.

    B. Bring hair to the front hairline, creating a ponytail, and secure with a rubber band. Squeeze and smooth the hair, creating a fan effect.

    C. Cut a straight horizontal line to the desired length. Release rubber band. **Caution: Hold hand over rubber band to prevent recoil action.**

    D. Beginning at the control axis, project the hair at 90 degrees elevation. Continue with subsections, checking and removing the points in the control zone.

    E. Comb hair into the natural fall distribution from the control axis of the head. Check and clean the outer perimeter baseline, customizing according to the desired results.

    F. Comb hair in a natural distribution towards the face, showing a soft and wispy line.

    G. Finished design.

8. Apply the liquid styling tool of choice to the hair.
9. Airform the hair to create the desired style.
10. Apply finishing spray to hold the completed style.
11. Follow standard clean-up procdures.
12. Document the Client Record/File.

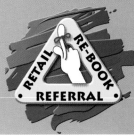

EVALUATION

GRADE

STUDENT'S NAME

ID#

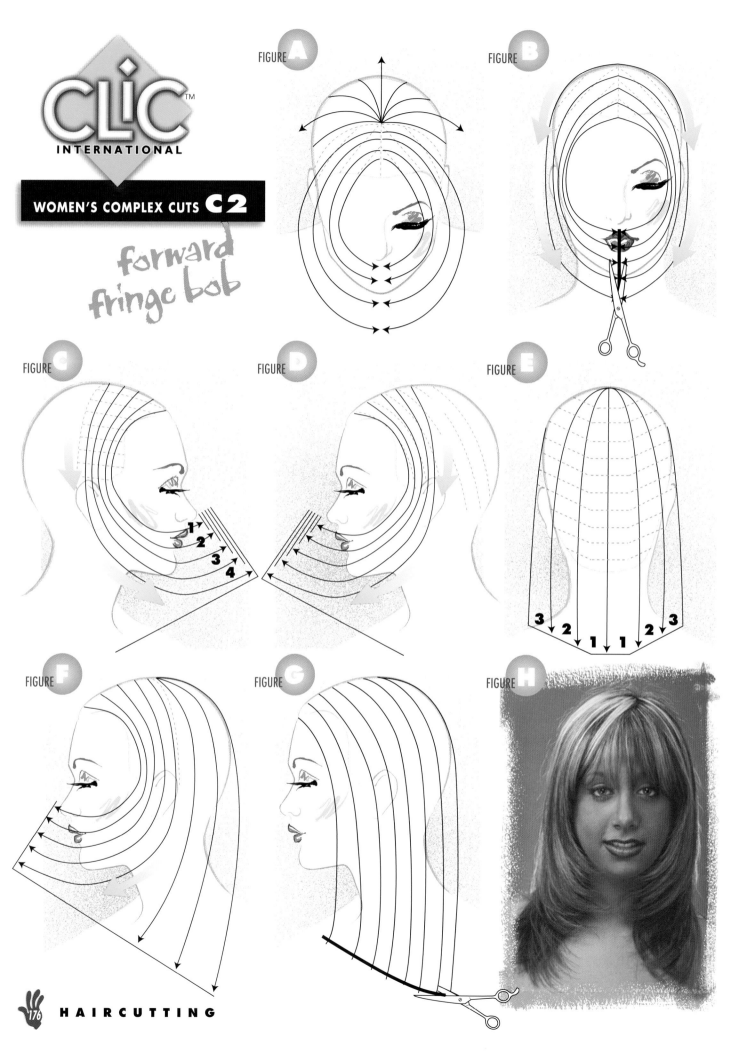

CLiC™
INTERNATIONAL

WOMEN'S COMPLEX CUTS **C2**

forward fringe bob

FIGURE A

FIGURE B

FIGURE C

FIGURE D

FIGURE E

FIGURE F

FIGURE G

FIGURE H

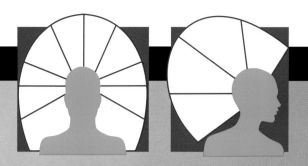

C2 forward fringe bob

OBJECTIVE

Master the FORWARD FRINGE BOB, a style that moves toward the face with short, caressing layers, yet still retains length in the back. It is a fringe cut in the front 1/3 (0.84cm) of the head and a negative elevation cut in the back 2/3 (1.7cm) of the head. The cut begins in the front 1/3 (0.84cm) of the head, with the longest lengths slightly below the chin. Texturizing may be added around front hairline areas.

TOOLS & MATERIALS

- Neck Strip
- Towels (2)
- Cape
- All-Purpose Brush
- Shampoo
- Shampoo Comb
- Conditioner
- Cutting Comb
- Clips or Clamps
- 5" (12.7 cm) or 6" (15.2 cm) Scissors
- Razor
- Styling Tool of Choice
- Liquid Styling Product
- Airformer
- Brushes
- Finishing Spray
- Client Record Card/File

PROCEDURE

"The Client Consultation is an important part of your professional service. Be sure to complete this step prior to each client service you provide. Your successful retail sales and customer satisfaction rates depend upon it!"

1. Drape the client in preparation for the service.
2. Thoroughly brush the client's hair to remove knots, tangles and hairspray.
3. Cleanse the hair with shampoo. Rinse thoroughly and shampoo again. Rinse.
4. Apply the appropriate conditioning product for the client's needs. Rinse thoroughly and towel dry.
5. Comb the hair to remove tangles.
6. Section the hair for the FORWARD FRINGE BOB and secure it with clips.
7. Perform the haircut as follows:
   A. Divide the head into the front 1/3 (0.84cm) and back 2/3 (1.7cm). The figure shows the correct distribution of hair from the partings.
   B. Using the center part as a point of reference, part diagonal lines toward the hairline. Direct each vertical plane close to the head and down toward the ear, then curve to the center of the face. Next, cut a vertical baseline from the top of the lip to below the chin.
   C. Direct each vertical plane slightly lower and slightly farther past the nose than the last one. This will continue the vertical baseline, creating

slightly longer lengths toward the bottom of the haircut.
   D. Continue the cut on the opposite side.
   E. Distribute the back 2/3 (1.7cm) of the head in vertical planes, as shown. Cut the back 2/3 (1.7cm) of the head with negative elevation. Begin by cutting the center plane with a horizontal baseline slightly below the mannequin base. Continue cutting from the center plane to the sides with a diagonal back baseline. Hair will gradually get shorter toward the front, connecting with the longest lengths in the front.
   F. Connect the diagonal back baseline with the lengths in the front.
   G. Distribute hair according to its natural fall. Check and clean the outer baseline.
   H. Finished design.
8. Apply the liquid styling tool of choice to the hair.
9. Airform the hair to create the desired style.
10. Apply finishing spray to hold the completed style.
11. Follow standard clean-up procedures.
12. Document the Client Record/File.

EVALUATION

GRADE

STUDENT'S NAME

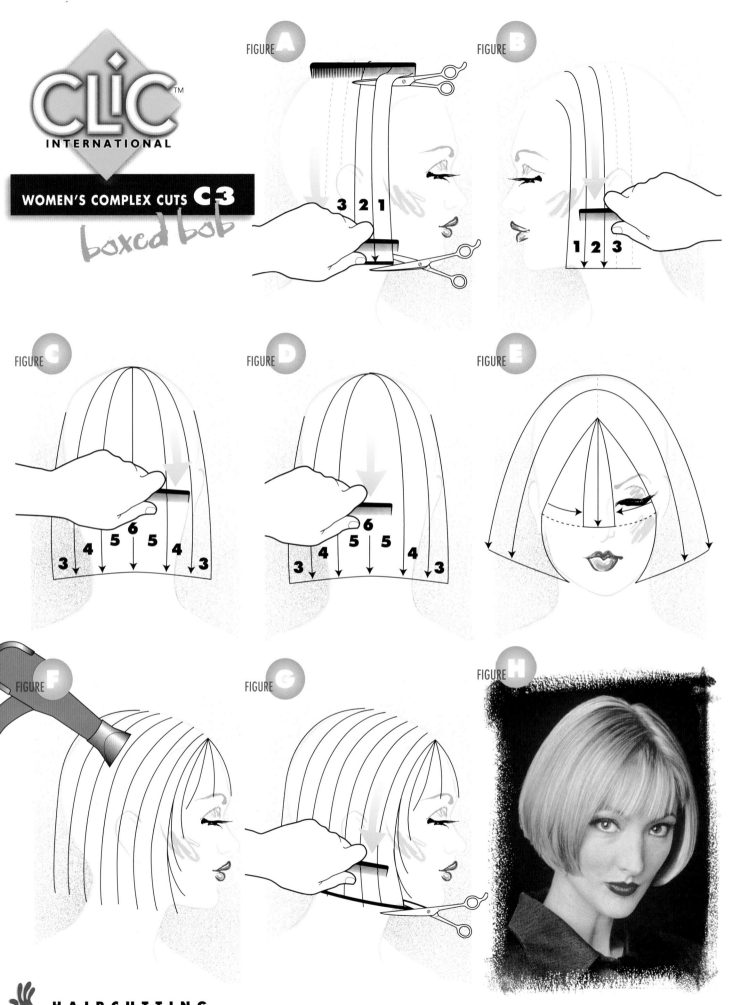

CLiC™
INTERNATIONAL

WOMEN'S COMPLEX CUTS **C-3**

boxed bob

FIGURE **A**

3 2 1

FIGURE **B**

1 2 3

FIGURE **C**

3 4 5 6 5 4 3

FIGURE **D**

3 4 5 6 5 4 3

FIGURE **E**

FIGURE **F**

FIGURE **G**

FIGURE **H**

C-3 boxed bob

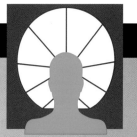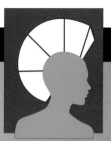

OBJECTIVE

Cut the BOXED BOB, a cut that derives its style from simplicity. This is a negative elevation short bob with a beveled baseline. The baseline is cut at the bottom of the chin. The hair is cut with a slight bevel, using a no-tension speed cut technique with scissors.

TOOLS & MATERIALS

- Neck Strip
- Towels (2)
- Cape
- All-Purpose Brush
- Shampoo
- Shampoo Comb
- Conditioner
- Cutting Comb
- Clips or Clamps
- Standard 5" (12.7 cm) Scissors
- Texturizing Tool of Choice
- Liquid Styling Product
- Airformer
- Brushes
- Finishing Spray
- Client Record Card/File

PROCEDURE

"The Client Consultation is an important part of your professional service. Be sure to complete this step prior to each client service you provide. Your successful retail sales and customer satisfaction rates depend upon it!"

1. Drape the client in preparation for the service.
2. Thoroughly brush the client's hair to remove knots, tangles and hairspray.
3. Cleanse the hair with shampoo. Rinse thoroughly and shampoo again. Rinse.
4. Apply the appropriate conditioning product for the client's needs. Rinse thoroughly and towel dry.
5. Comb the hair to remove tangles.
6. Section the hair for the BOXED BOB and secure it with clips.
7. Perform the haircut as follows:
A. Comb hair from the volume zone to the indentation zone. Using vertical lines, section a 1/3 (0.84cm) portion and break it down into thirds. Start at plane #1 and work back to the ear. Place comb at part line at the top of the head. Using scissors, slightly lift and lock in teeth of comb. Pull comb and scissors down to the rim zone. Pull scissors out and continue projecting hair slightly from the head. Then,slightly turn spine of comb to a 45 degrees angle with teeth positioned on scalp.
B. Continue to cut using comb and scissors technique with no tension on both sides.

C-D: Cut the back indentation zone with a beveled edge and use negative elevation. Begin on the sides and work toward the center plane. Cut a horizontal baseline using the comb and scissors technique. Work from side to center, matching the length and holding comb and scissors at a 45 degree angle at the baseline.
E. Cut the bang area using a speed cutting technique. Section off a triangular area at the outer edge of each eye and connect approximately 2" (5.1cm) back from the center hairline or at the end of the frontal bone. Hold all hair to the middle and squeeze cut with tension to just above the tip of the nose. This will create a curved bang.
F. Using the slide technique, soften the outer edges, framing the face. Using an airformer, dry the hair into a straight design.
G. Check and re-cut hair using a no-tension technique.
H. Finished design.
8. Apply the liquid styling tool of choice to the hair.
9. Airform the hair to create the desired style.
10. Apply finishing spray to hold the completed style.
11. Follow standard clean-up procedures.
12. Document the Client Record/File.

EVALUATION

_____

_____

GRADE

_____

_____
STUDENT'S NAME

_____
ID#

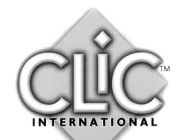

disrupted bob

FIGURE **A**

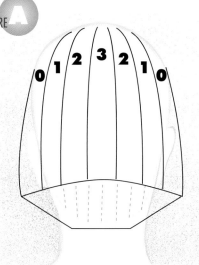

0 1 2 3 2 1 0

FIGURE **B**

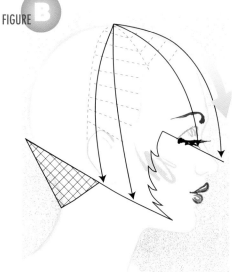

FIGURE **C**

4"

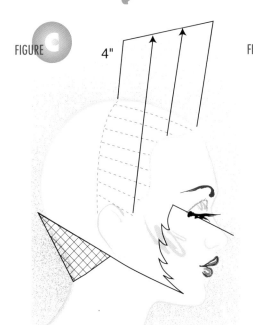

FIGURE **D**

1 2 3 2 1

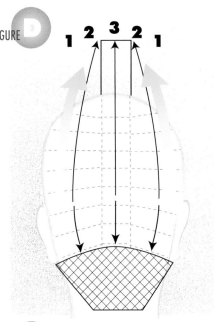

FIGURE **E**

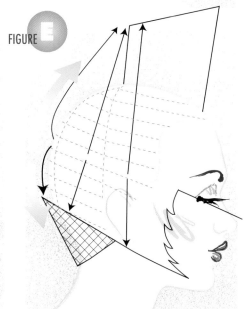

FIGURE **F**

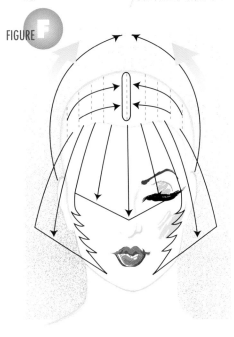

FIGURE **G**

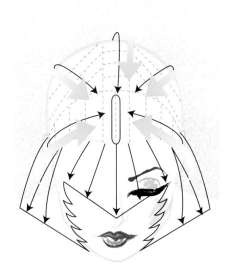

FIGURE **H**

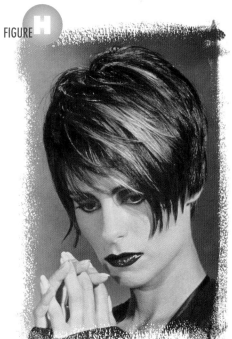

C4 disrupted bob

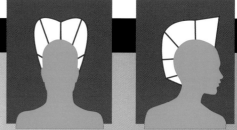

OBJECTIVE

Learn to cut the DISRUPTED BOB, an uncontrived short cut with a close-fitting back. This cut is created by using a squeeze cutting technique and also uses a slide cutting technique to blend the bang area to the bottom baseline in order to create softness in the frontal perimeter.

TOOLS & MATERIALS

- Neck Strip
- Towels (2)
- Cape
- All-Purpose Brush
- Shampoo
- Shampoo Comb
- Conditioner
- Cutting Comb
- Clips or Clamps
- Razor
- Standard 5" (12.7 cm) Scissors
- Texturizing Tool of Choice
- Liquid Styling Product
- Airformer
- Brushes
- Finishing Spray
- Client Record Card/File

PROCEDURE

"The Client Consultation is an important part of your professional service. Be sure to complete this step prior to each client service you provide. Your successful retail sales and customer satisfaction rates depend upon it!"

1. Drape the client in preparation for the service.
2. Thoroughly brush the client's hair to remove knots, tangles and hairspray.
3. Cleanse the hair with shampoo. Rinse thoroughly and shampoo again. Rinse.
4. Apply the appropriate conditioning product for the client's needs. Rinse thoroughly and towel dry.
5. Comb the hair to remove tangles.
6. Section the hair for the DISRUPTED BOB and secure it with clips.
7. Perform the haircut as follows:
   A. Starting in the indentation zone, create an inverted diagonal section in the occipital area. Use a speed cutting technique to create the weight line. Begin with the center plane and squeeze the entire component up to the top of the inverted diagonal section. Cut the hair in an inverted diagonal line with a forward motion using three- (3) finger elevation at the base of the occipital bone. Continue cutting the weight line, working from the center to the side and reducing your finger elevation as indicated in each plane. Complete the area by customizing your perimeter baseline to create the desired result.
   B. Separate the bang area from the sides. Continue the diagonal forward movement from the side baseline toward the middle of the chin. Cut the entire side using tension with negative elevation. Use a diagonal line from the corner of the eye to the tip of the nose to the bang area. This is cut with negative elevation in its natural fall distribution. Carve a "C" shaping to blend the bang to the hanging length at the sides. Use slide cutting to soften the perimeter weight. With the hair held close to the face, begin at the corner of the eye and slide down the strand toward the mouth.
   C. Cut the anti-head guideline 4" (10.2 cm) at the control axis and blend to the longest lengths at the hairline. Create layering by using horizontal lines and directing all lengths up to the interior guide area and cut.
   D. Divide the back into three (3) panels using the control axis as a guide. Using positive elevation and a stationary guideline, bring up all of panel #3 and cut with a squeeze cutting technique. The outside borders of #3 become the guidelines for panels #2 and #1.
   E. Blend the disrupted layering by cutting the portion from the side to the center back panel.
   F. Check and blend all perimeter and interior lines.
   G. Check and blend all areas from front to back.
   H. Finished design.
8. Apply the liquid styling tool of choice to the hair.
9. Airform the hair to create the desired style.
10. Apply finishing spray to hold the completed style.
11. Follow standard clean-up procedures.
12. Document the Client Record/File.

EVALUATION

GRADE

STUDENT'S NAME

ID#

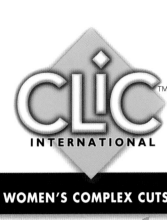

WOMEN'S COMPLEX CUTS **C5**

asymmetrical

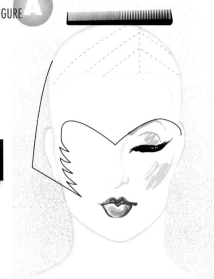

FIGURE B

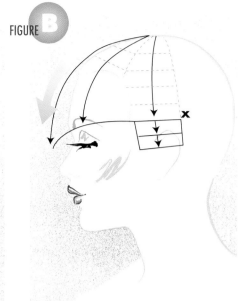

FIGURE C

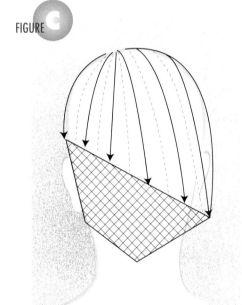

FIGURE D

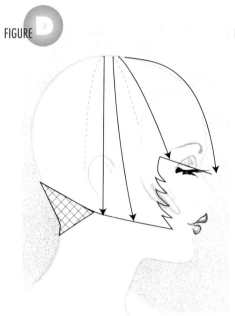

FIGURE E   3"

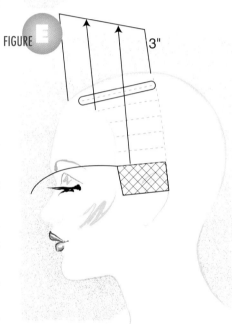

FIGURE F   3"

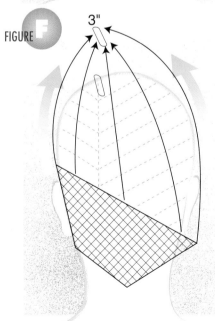

FIGURE G

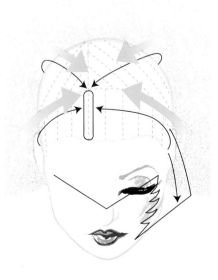

FIGURE H

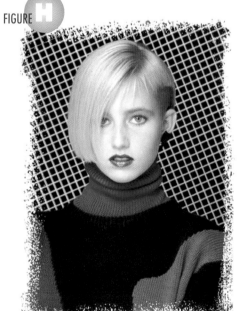

C5 asymmetrical

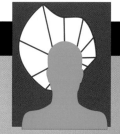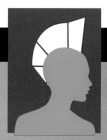

OBJECTIVE

Craft an ASYMMETRICAL cut, a convertible style that can look asymmetric or symmetric depending upon the partings used to style the hair. It is cut short on one side with a diagonal weight line from the short side around the back to just below the ear on the long side.

TOOLS & MATERIALS

- Neck Strip
- Towels (2)
- Cape
- All-Purpose Brush
- Shampoo
- Shampoo Comb
- Conditioner
- Cutting Comb
- Clips or Clamps
- Standard 5" (12.7 cm) Scissors
- Clippers
- Razor
- Texturizing Tool of Choice
- Liquid Styling Product
- Airformer
- Brushes
- Finishing Spray
- Client Record Card/File

PROCEDURE

"The Client Consultation is an important part of your professional service. Be sure to complete this step prior to each client service you provide. Your successful retail sales and customer satisfaction rates depend upon it!"

1. Drape the client in preparation for the service.
2. Thoroughly brush the client's hair to remove knots, tangles and hairspray.
3. Cleanse the hair with shampoo. Rinse thoroughly and shampoo again. Rinse.
4. Apply the appropriate conditioning product for the client's needs. Rinse thoroughly and towel dry.
5. Comb the hair to remove tangles.
6. Section the hair for the ASYMMETRICAL and secure it with clips.
7. Perform the haircut as follows:

   A. Use an off-center part to create the asymmetrical design. Place a comb flat on the top of the head at the control zone. Create a front-to-back part from the point where the comb leaves the head on the left side.

   B. Begin the cut on the short side of the head. Separate the bang area from the sides. Cut a horizontal plane using one-(1) finger elevation. Cut all hair from the volume zone at one- (1) finger elevation to the second guideline (X). Cut the bang with negative elevation, blending from the weight line to the center of the nose.

   C. In the back, blend the diagonal weight line from the front weight line to the bottom of the left ear. Work around to the long side of the head using two- (2) finger elevation. Tension comb all hair smoothly in its natural fall distribution. Cut hair below the weight line using a traveling guide from a two- (2) finger elevation to a one- (1) finger elevation.

   D. The weight line on the heavy side extends from the weight line in the back, level with the mouth. Speed cut all hair using negative elevation. Cut the bang area negative in its natural fall distribution, removing 1/4" (0.6 cm).

   E. Create a line parted at the off-center parting of the frontal volume zone. Cut this guideline anti-head from 3" (7.6 cm) at the control zone to the longest lengths in the bang area. Bring hair on both sides of the head straight up to a stationary guide and cut using horizontal partings. Use a squeeze cutting technique.

   F. Extend the off-center guide to the back of the head, blending from 3" (7.6 cm) at the control zone to the longest lengths in the weight line area. Bring all hair straight up to this point using the squeeze cutting technique. Use diagonal partings in the back of the head.

   G. Blend the volume and indentation zones. Carve a "C" shaping into the bang on the short side of the head to create shorter lengths for the bang area. Texturize with a razor, using a backcombing technique. Hold the razor on a slight angle to the strand in order to remove the desired amount of bulk. Use the rolling razor technique in the nape to soften the ends.

   H. Finished design.

8. Apply the liquid styling tool of choice to the hair.
9. Airform the hair to create the desired style.
10. Apply finishing spray to hold the completed style.
11. Follow standard clean-up procedures.
12. Document the Client Record/File.

EVALUATION

GRADE

STUDENT'S NAME

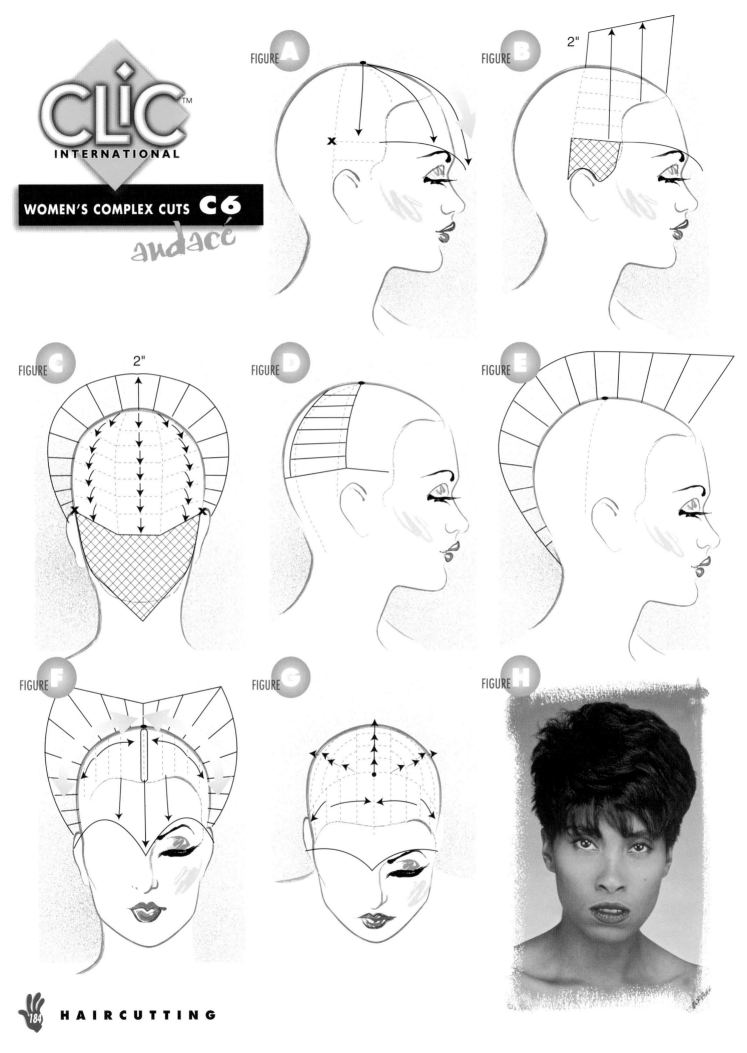

CLiC™
INTERNATIONAL

WOMEN'S COMPLEX CUTS **C6**

audacé

FIGURE A

FIGURE B   2"

FIGURE C   2"

FIGURE D

FIGURE E

FIGURE F

FIGURE G

FIGURE H

x

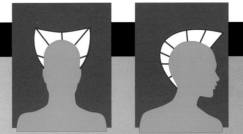

C6 audacé

OBJECTIVE

Master the AUDACÉ cut, a short, tapered cut with longer lengths for softness in the front. The front of the head is cut anti-head, creating the longest lengths in the bang area.

TOOLS & MATERIALS

- Neck Strip
- Towels (2)
- Cape
- All-Purpose Brush
- Shampoo
- Shampoo Comb
- Conditioner
- Cutting Comb
- Clips or Clamps
- Standard 5" (12.7 cm) Scissors
- Liquid Styling Product
- Airformer
- Brushes
- Finishing Spray
- Client Record Card/File

PROCEDURE

"The Client Consultation is an important part of your professional service. Be sure to complete this step prior to each client service you provide. Your successful retail sales and customer satisfaction rates depend upon it!"

1. Drape the client in preparation for the service.
2. Thoroughly brush the client's hair to remove knots, tangles and hairspray.
3. Cleanse the hair with shampoo. Rinse thoroughly and shampoo again. Rinse.
4. Apply the appropriate conditioning product for the client's needs. Rinse thoroughly and towel dry.
5. Comb the hair to remove tangles.
6. Section the hair for the AUDACÉ and secure it with clips.
7. Perform the haircut as follows:
   A. Cut the indentation zone using a traveling guide for the first two planes or subsections. Cut the indentation zones of the first and second subsections using one - (1) finger elevation. Comb down all hair above the second plane and cut to the second subsection, at the rim line, creating a weight line (X). Cut the bang negatively, blending from the weight line to the center of the nose. Carve a "C" shaping into the side of the bang. Repeat on the other side.
   B. Cut a center guideline on top of the head from the control axis. Cut the guideline, blending from 2 1/2" (6.4cm) at the control axis to the longest lengths at the nose. Bring the sides straight up from the indentation zone to the control axis in the volume zone. Repeat on opposite side.
   C. Cut the nape area to just above the ears using one - (1) finger elevation with positive elevation and horizontal

lines. Re-cut the bottom baseline around the ear to a clean line. The volume zone of the back is divided into three (3) panels. Beginning at the control axis, cut the center panel. Using a traveling guide, work down toward the indentation zone. Using the 2 1/2" (6.4 cm) guide at the control axis, perform a radial cut using a traveling guide. Project the hair at 90 degrees positive elevation, gradually decrease the length and blend with the lengths in the nape. Cut the side sections in the same manner, blending the lengths in the front and center back. The lengths in the front are longer than the lengths in the back. **Do not remove this extra length**, as this area is cut to blend the front and back only.

   D. Cut the lengths in the side back sections to blend with the front and back area.
   E. Blend and check all lengths in the back of the head.
   F. Blend and check all lengths in the front of the head. The weight line, indicated by the longer lengths, should remain.
   G. Blend and check baseline in the natural fall distribution.
   H. Finished design.
8. Apply the liquid styling tool of choice to the hair.
9. Airform the hair to create the desired style.
10. Apply finishing spray to hold the completed style.
11. Follow standard clean-up procedures.
12. Document the Client Record/File.

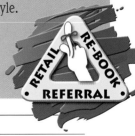

EVALUATION

GRADE

STUDENT'S NAME

ID#

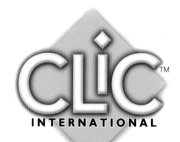

WOMEN'S COMPLEX CUTS C7

clipette cut

FIGURE **A**

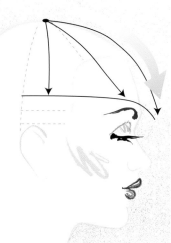

FIGURE **B**

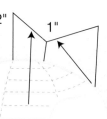
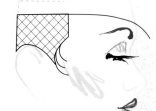

2" 1"

FIGURE **C**

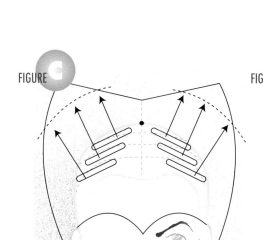

FIGURE **D**

2"

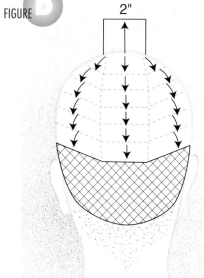

FIGURE **E**

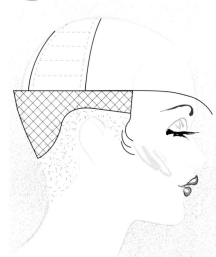

FIGURE **F**

2"
1" 2"

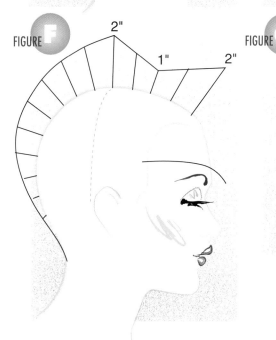

FIGURE **G**

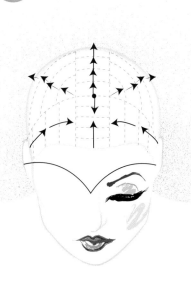

FIGURE **H**

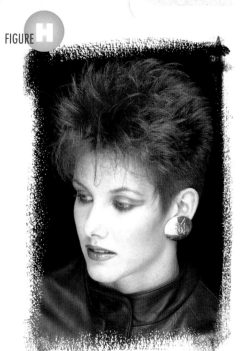

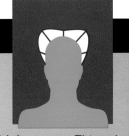
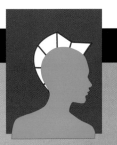

C7 clippette

OBJECTIVE

Learn the CLIPPETTE, a finger-dried, wash'n'wear cut. This style is cut short to long, moving up the head using clipper and comb control in the indentation zone. The front of the head is cut anti-head with the shortest lengths at the back of the frontal plane.

TOOLS & MATERIALS

- Neck Strip
- Towels (2)
- Cape
- All-Purpose Brush
- Shampoo
- Shampoo Comb
- Conditioner
- Cutting Comb
- Clips or Clamps
- Standard 5" (12.7 cm) Scissors
- Razor
- Clippers
- Texturizing Tool of Choice
- Liquid Styling Product
- Airformer
- Brushes
- Finishing Spray
- Client Record Card/File

PROCEDURE

"The Client Consultation is an important part of your professional service. Be sure to complete this step prior to each client service you provide. Your successful retail sales and customer satisfaction rates depend upon it!"

1. Drape the client in preparation for the service.
2. Thoroughly brush the client's hair to remove knots, tangles and hairspray.
3. Cleanse the hair with shampoo. Rinse thoroughly and shampoo again. Rinse.
4. Apply the appropriate conditioning product for the client's needs. Rinse thoroughly and towel dry.
5. Comb the hair to remove tangles.
6. Section the hair for the CLIPPETTE and secure it with clips.
7. Perform the haircut as follows:

   A. Divide the frontal plane from the front 1/3 (0.84cm). Cut the indentation zone of the sides with comb and clipper control. Comb down all hair in the volume zone and cut to the rim line. Cut the bang, blending from the weight line to just above the bridge of the nose.

   B. Cut a center line from 1" (2.5 cm) behind the frontal plane to 2" (5.1 cm) at the control axis. Bring up all side hair from the volume zone and cut to this guide. Cut the bang area by blending from the longest length at the hairline to 1" (2.5 cm) at the back of the frontal plane. Bring up all lengths in this section and cut to this guideline.

   C. Part vertical planes in the blending area between the volume and indentation zones. Positively project hair in each plane and remove the corner to create softness.

   D. Radial cut the indentation zone of the back using comb control. Divide the volume zone into three (3) panels. Cut the center section first using clipper and comb control. Use positive elevation from the length of the rim to the control zone, approximately 2" (5.1 cm).

   E. Cut the side sections of the back in the same manner, blending the longer lengths in the front of the head and the shorter lengths in the center back.

   F. Check and blend all lengths from the indentation to the volume zones.

   G. Check the finished haircut in its natural fall direction.

   H. Finished design.

8. Apply the liquid styling tool of choice to the hair.
9. Airform the hair to create the desired style.
10. Apply finishing spray to hold the completed style.
11. Follow standard clean-up procedures.
12. Document the Client Record/File.

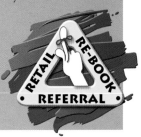

EVALUATION

GRADE

STUDENT'S NAME

ID#

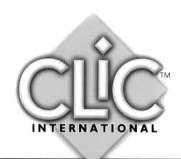

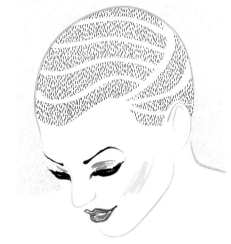

FIGURE **C**

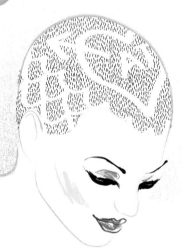

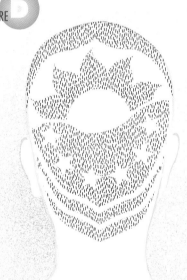

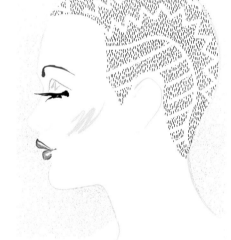

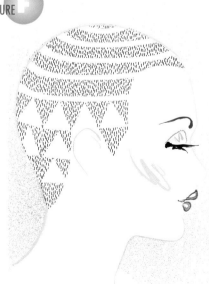

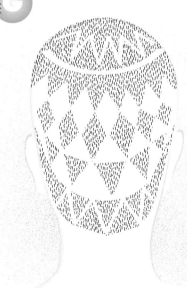

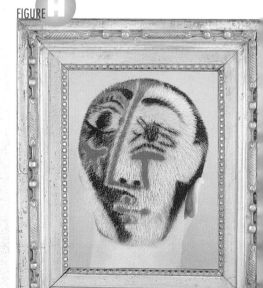

Creative Clipper cuts first became popular in the 1970s as a component of the stylish street fashions worn by the trendsetters of that generation. Today this inventiveness is displayed in creations ranging from simple to complex in design.

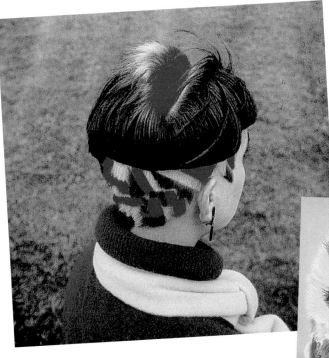

This is your opportunity to give it a try! Use our examples, or better yet, create your own artistic clipper creation. Remember: there are no rules. Let your imagination be your guide!

Cut and color your design to make a strong visual impact with your creation!

NOTES

_____

_____

_____

_____

_____

_____

_____

_____

_____

_____

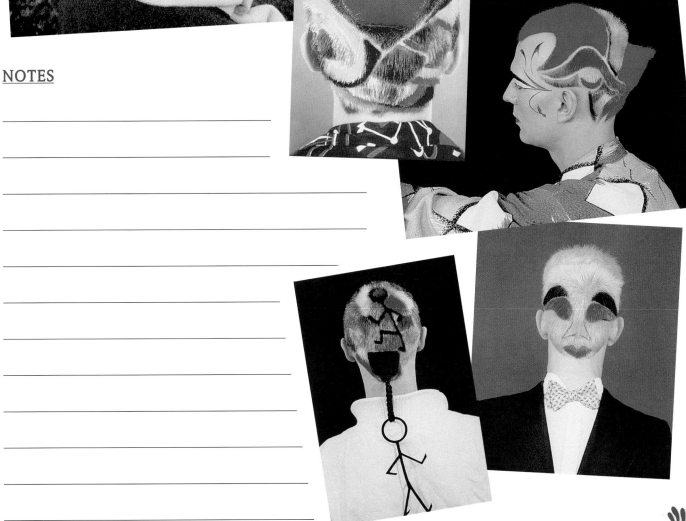

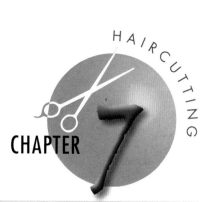

crew cut

square beard

men's **renegade** wedge

flat top

shadow beard

CHAPTER 7

HAIRCUTTING

Art of Haircutting

MEN'S CUTS

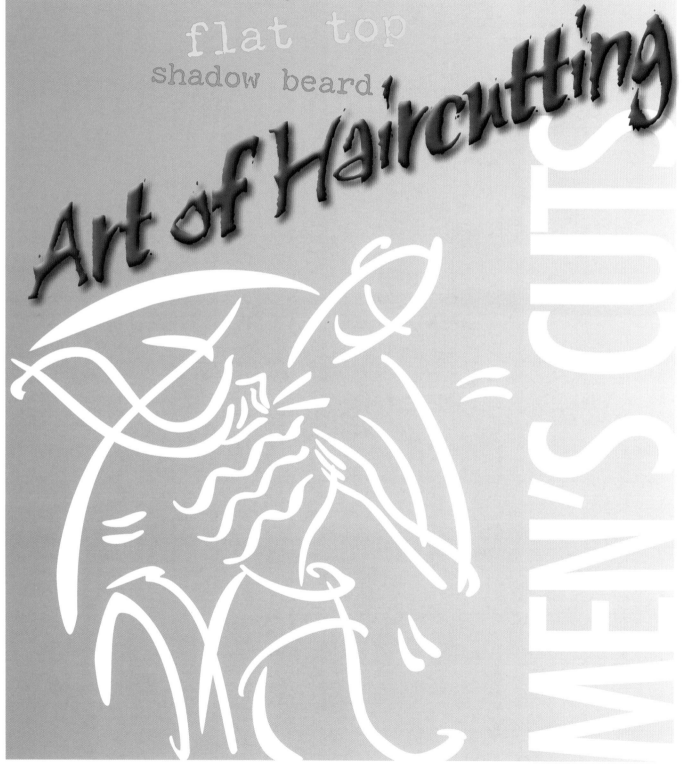

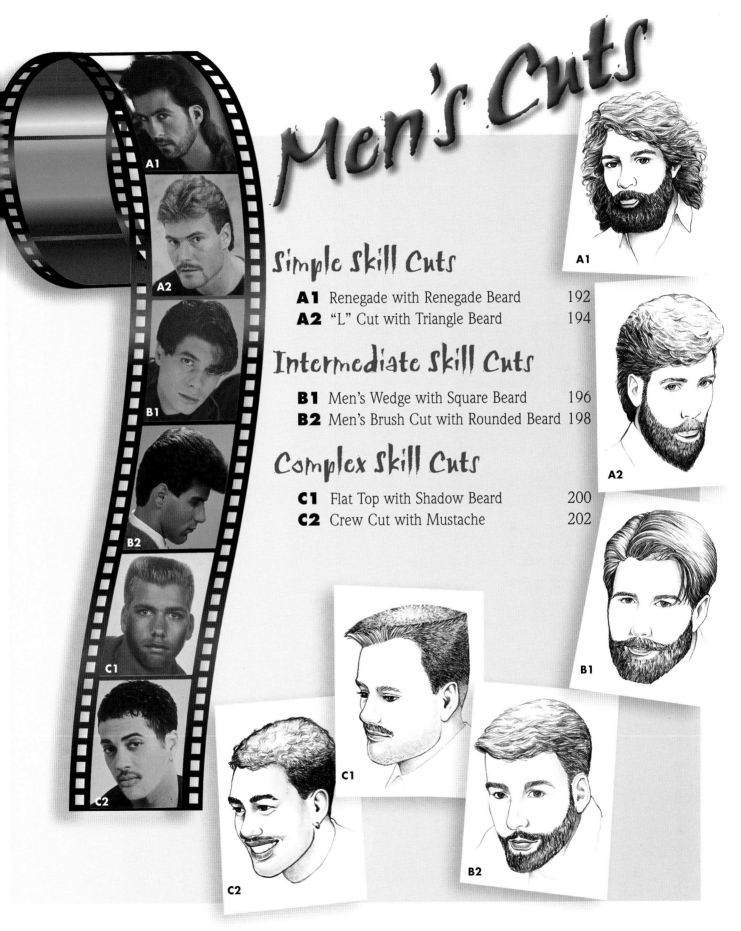

Men's Cuts

Simple Skill Cuts

Intermediate Skill Cuts

Complex Skill Cuts

A1

A2

B1

B2

C1

C2

A1

A2

B1

B2

C1

C2

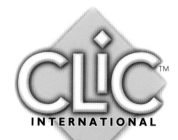

MEN'S SIMPLE CUTS **A 1**

renegade with renegade beard

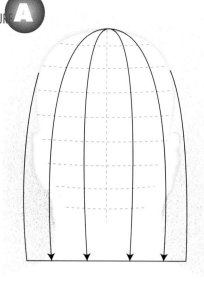

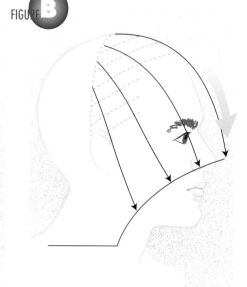

FIGURE **C**
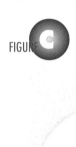
6"
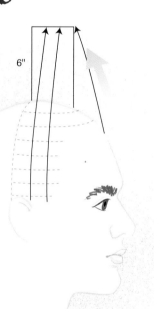

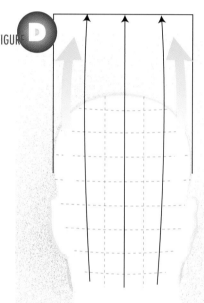

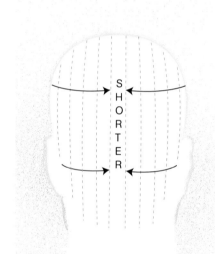

SHORTER

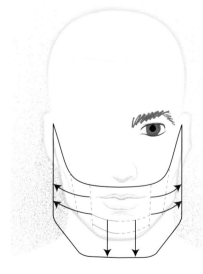

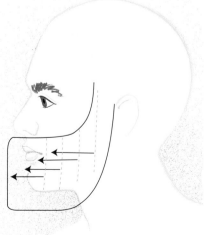

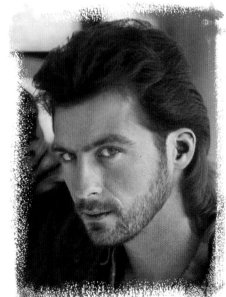

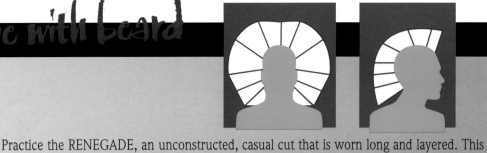

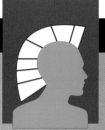

A1 renegade with beard

OBJECTIVE

Practice the RENEGADE, an unconstructed, casual cut that is worn long and layered. This is a reverse positive elevation layered haircut with many new variations. The renegade beard is a full beard to help balance the haircut.

TOOLS & MATERIALS

- Neck Strip
- Towels (2)
- Cape
- All-Purpose Brush
- Shampoo
- Shampoo Comb
- Conditioner
- Cutting Comb
- Clips or Clamps
- Trimmer
- Standard 5" (12.7 cm) or 6" (15.2 cm) Scissors
- Texturizing Tool of Choice
- Liquid Styling Product
- Airformer
- Brushes
- Finishing Spray
- Client Record Card/File

PROCEDURE

"The Client Consultation is an important part of your professional service. Be sure to complete this step prior to each client service you provide. Your successful retail sales and customer satisfaction rates depend upon it!"

1. Drape the client in preparation for the service.
2. Thoroughly brush the client's hair to remove knots, tangles and hairspray.
3. Cleanse the hair with shampoo. Rinse thoroughly and shampoo again. Rinse.
4. Apply the appropriate conditioning product for the client's needs. Rinse thoroughly and towel dry.
5. Comb the hair to remove tangles.
6. Section the hair for the RENEGADE and secure it with clips/clamps.
7. Perform the haircut as follows:

   A. Cut the back baseline in a straight horizontal line. Take horizontal partings and cut parallel to the baseline.

   B. Cut the front baseline on a diagonal from the tip of the nose to the established length at the ear. Part the hair parallel to the baseline and shift it forward to blend. Shift less above the ear to blend with the back lengths.

   C. Create reverse positive elevation in the front of the head by establishing a 6" (15.2 cm) guide on the top of the head. Bring all hair up and cut using the squeeze technique. Using horizontal partings, shift the frontal area back slightly to create more length. Repeat on the opposite side.

   D. Divide the back of the head into three (3) panels. Cut the center panel first, using a 6" (15.2 cm) stationary guide from the control axis. Bring up all

hair in this panel and use a squeeze technique. Cut the two (2) side panels in the same manner using the squeeze technique.

   E. To create shorter hair in the center back, use a vertical section to cut and blend the top lengths to the bottom. Weight must be maintained in the nape. Using vertical planes, bring hair on both sides of this guide to the center and apply a squeeze technique.

   F. Cut the length of the beard approximately 1" (2.5 cm) above the bottom of the neck. Bring all beard hair down to this guide and cut with negative elevation. Create the side beard by blending length and using the squeeze technique from the ear down to the side of the bottom neck area.

   G. Reduce bulk by parting a vertical plane in the center from the base of the beard. Cut a straight vertical guide using the bottom baseline as a guide. Remember to leave weight at the perimeter. Cut vertical planes while moving from the center to the sides and use a portion of the previously cut vertical section as a guide.

   H. Finished design with beard.

8. Apply the liquid styling tool of choice to the hair.
9. Airform the hair to create the desired style.
10. Apply finishing spray to hold the completed style.
11. Follow standard clean-up procedures.
12. Document the Client Record/File.

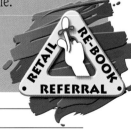

EVALUATION

GRADE

STUDENT'S NAME

ID#

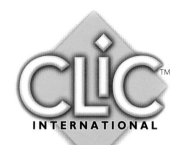

MEN'S SIMPLE CUTS A2

"L" cut with triangle beard

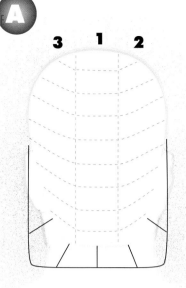

FIGURE A

3 1 2

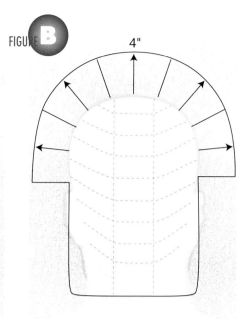

FIGURE B

4"

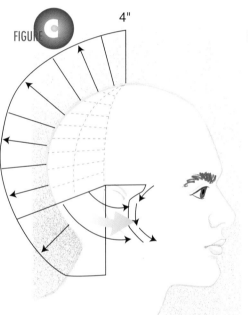

FIGURE C

4"

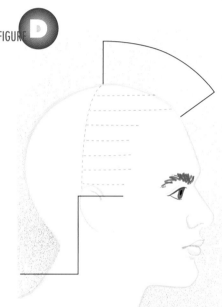

FIGURE D

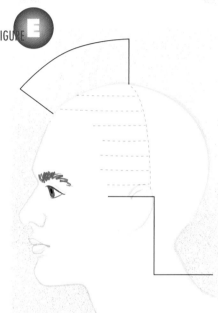

FIGURE E

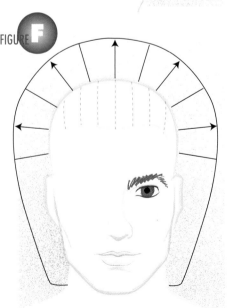

FIGURE F

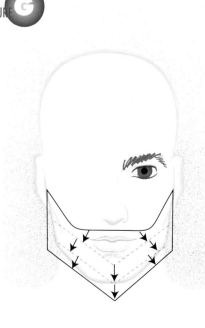

FIGURE G

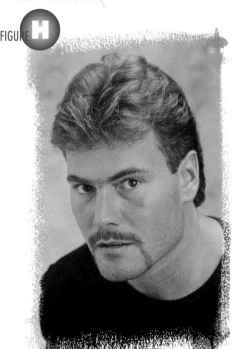

FIGURE H

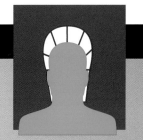
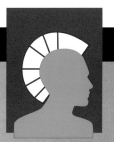

OBJECTIVE

Learn to create the "L" CUT, a versatile look with longer length in the back of the head and shorter length in the frontal area of the head. This style is a radial layered haircut that utilizes a scissors and razor. The Triangle Beard has a well-defined "V" baseline.

TOOLS & MATERIALS

- Neck Strip
- Towels (2)
- Cape
- All-Purpose Brush
- Shampoo
- Shampoo Comb
- Conditioner
- Cutting Comb
- Clips
- Trimmer
- Standard 5" (12.7 cm) or 6" (15.2 cm) Scissors
- Texturizing Tool of Choice
- Liquid Styling Product
- Airformer
- Brushes
- Finishing Spray
- Client Record Card/File

PROCEDURE

"The Client Consultation is an important part of your professional service. Be sure to complete this step prior to each client service you provide. Your successful retail sales and customer satisfaction rates depend upon it!"

1. Drape the client in preparation for the service.
2. Thoroughly brush the client's hair to remove knots, tangles and hairspray.
3. Cleanse the hair with shampoo. Rinse thoroughly and shampoo again. Rinse.
4. Apply the appropriate conditioning product for the client's needs. Rinse thoroughly and towel dry.
5. Comb the hair to remove tangles.
6. Section the hair for the "L" CUT and secure it with clips.
7. Perform the haircut as follows:

   A. Divide the back of the head into three (3) panels. Cut a horizontal baseline at collar length. Make all partings parallel to the baseline. Begin cutting in the center and move to each side. Cut the hair using positive elevation with vertical lines.

   B. Using positive elevation, raise the hair above the ears at 90 degrees to create a completely rounded shape throughout the back.

   C. Cut the entire back of the head vertically from the indentation zone to the control zone. Pull the hair directly behind the ear forward and cut in a curved shape.

   D. Cut the front baseline, blending from the tip of the nose to the baseline already established at the ear. Cut the side using a positive elevation of 90 degrees to blend the frontal area to the indentation zone in the nape.

   E. Repeat the same technique on the other side.

   F. Cut the entire head using vertical lines throughout.

   G. Create the Triangle Beard by cutting a diagonal front line on both sides and forming a center point. Cut the baseline at negative elevation, for a "V" shape. Create all partings parallel to the baseline.

   H. Finished design with beard.

8. Apply the liquid styling tool of choice to the hair.
9. Airform the hair to create the desired style.
10. Apply finishing spray to hold the completed style.
11. Follow standard clean-up procedures.
12. Document the Client Record/File.

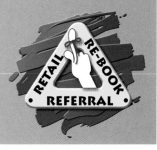

EVALUATION

GRADE

STUDENT'S NAME

ID#

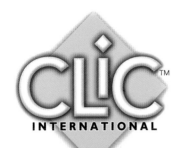

MEN'S INTERMEDIATE CUTS B1

men's wedge with square beard

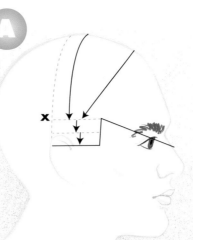

x

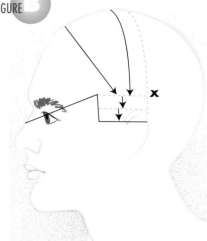

x

FIGURE C

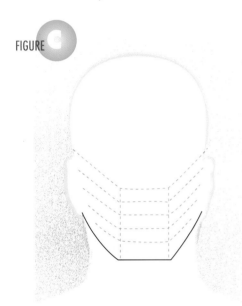

FIGURE D

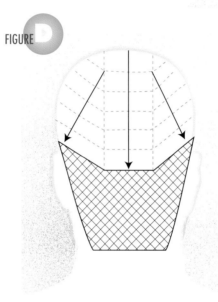

FIGURE E

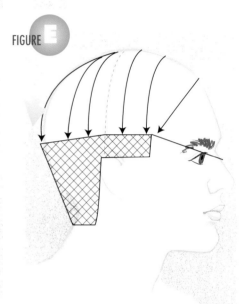

FIGURE F

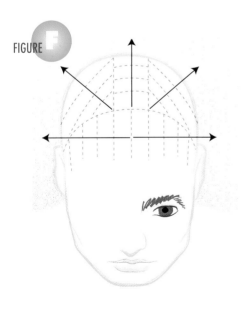

FIGURE G

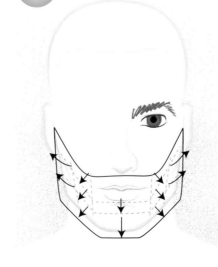

FIGURE H

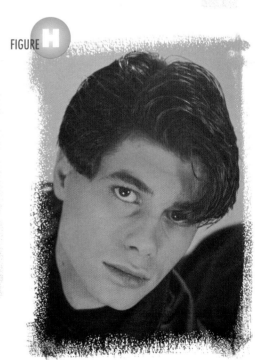

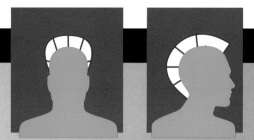

B1 men's wedge with beard

OBJECTIVE

Construct the MEN'S WEDGE. This graduated, short style is cut close on the sides and nape and longer in the crown area, giving hair mobility and producing a soft weight line. This positive elevation haircut is created using a scissors and clipper. The square beard complements the weight created in the haircut.

TOOLS & MATERIALS

- Neck Strip
- Towels (2)
- Cape
- All-Purpose Brush
- Shampoo
- Shampoo Comb
- Conditioner
- Cutting Comb
- Taper Comb
- Clips or Clamps
- Clipper
- Standard 5" (12.7 cm) or 6" (15.2 cm) Scissors
- Trimmer
- Texturizing Tool of Choice
- Liquid Styling Product
- Airformer
- Brushes
- Finishing Spray
- Client Record Card/File

PROCEDURE

"The Client Consultation is an important part of your professional service. Be sure to complete this step prior to each client service you provide. Your successful retail sales and customer satisfaction rates depend upon it!"

1. Drape the client in preparation for the service.
2. Thoroughly brush the client's hair to remove knots, tangles and hairspray.
3. Cleanse the hair with shampoo. Rinse thoroughly and shampoo again. Rinse.
4. Apply the appropriate conditioning product for the client's needs. Rinse thoroughly and towel dry.
5. Comb the hair to remove tangles.
6. Section the hair for the MEN'S WEDGE and secure it with clips.
7. Perform the haircut as follows:
   A. Cut a horizontal baseline at the top portion of the ear. Then cut the hair using a positive elevation 45 degree angle and horizontal partings in the indentation zone. Cut hair length down in the volume zone to the longest lengths in the indentation zone, creating a weight line (X). Shift hairline lengths back to create increased length toward the nose.
   B. Repeat on the other side of the head.
   C. Cut a horizontal baseline in the indentation zone 1" (2.5 cm) above the neck. Blend the diagonal sides of the baseline between the length at the ear and the nape. Cut the center section below the rim zone using positive elevation at 90 degrees and horizontal

   partings. Cut the side back sections by blending the positive elevation at the front with the layering in the center back.
   D. Create the weight line in the back of the head by bringing all lengths down from the volume zone to below the rim zone in a natural fall distribution. Positively elevate the stationary guide at a 45 degree angle.
   E. Use positive elevation to blend throughout the rim zone. Blend the weight line within the natural fall distribution. Shift back the hair in front to create increased length toward the nose.
   F. Check and blend all hair in its natural fall distribution.
   G. Cut a horizontal baseline from one corner of the mouth to the other. Cut a vertical baseline at the side, blending from the length at the ear. Blend a diagonal line between the ear and the corner of the mouth. Cut partings parallel to the bottom baseline at a positive elevation throughout the beard.
   H. Finished design with beard.
8. Apply the liquid styling tool of choice to the hair.
9. Airform the hair to create the desired style.
10. Apply finishing spray to hold the completed style.
11. Follow standard clean-up procedures.
12. Document the Client Record/File.

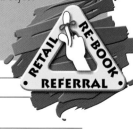

EVALUATION

GRADE

STUDENT'S NAME

ID#

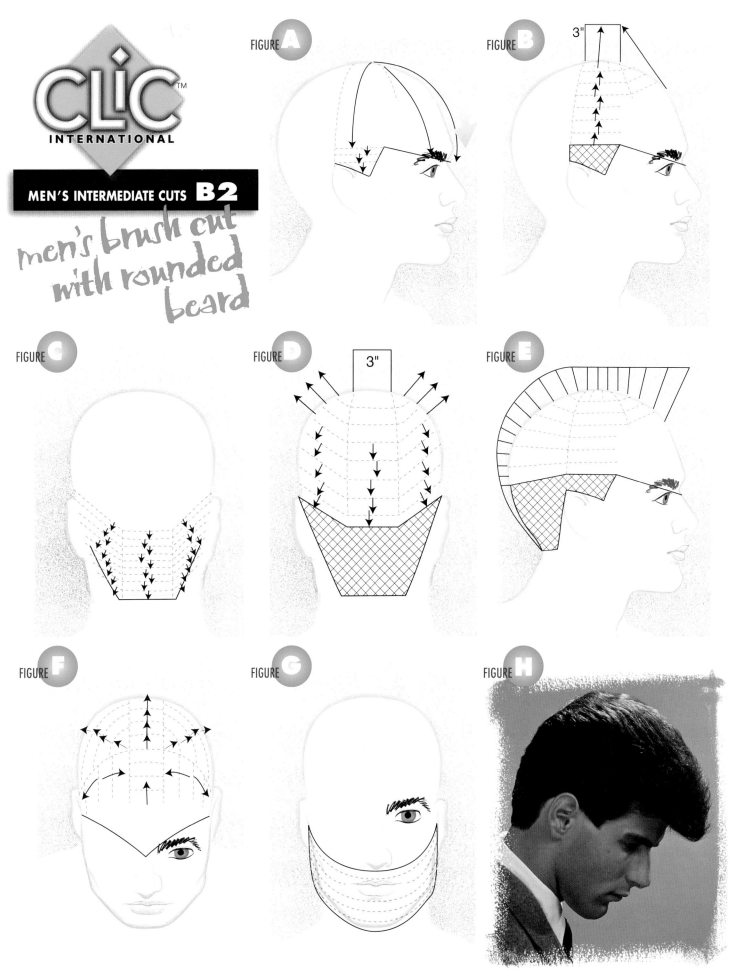

CLiC™
INTERNATIONAL

MEN'S INTERMEDIATE CUTS B2

men's brush cut
with rounded
beard

FIGURE A

FIGURE B
3"

FIGURE C

FIGURE D
3"

FIGURE E

FIGURE F

FIGURE G

FIGURE H

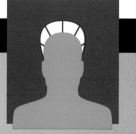
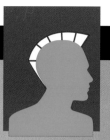

OBJECTIVE

Master the MEN'S BRUSH CUT, a versatile style that can be worn straight, curly or wavy. This short haircut consists of a positive tapered nape with longer lengths above the volume zone of the head. A weight area is cut just above the rim zone. A short rounded beard complements this cut.

TOOLS & MATERIALS

- Neck Strip
- Towels (2)
- Cape
- All-Purpose Brush
- Shampoo

- Shampoo Comb
- Conditioner
- Cutting Comb
- Taper Comb
- Clips

- Standard 5" (12.7 cm) or 6" (15.2 cm) Scissors
- Trimmer
- Razor
- Liquid Styling Product

- Airformer
- Brushes
- Finishing Spray
- Client Record Card/File

PROCEDURE

"The Client Consultation is an important part of your professional service. Be sure to complete this step prior to each client service you provide. Your successful retail sales and customer satisfaction rates depend upon it!"

1. Drape the client in preparation for the service.
2. Thoroughly brush the client's hair to remove knots, tangles and hairspray.
3. Cleanse the hair with shampoo. Rinse thoroughly and shampoo again. Rinse.
4. Apply the appropriate conditioning product for the client's needs. Rinse thoroughly and towel dry.
5. Comb the hair to remove tangles.
6. Section the hair for the MEN'S BRUSH CUT and secure it with clips.
7. Perform the haircut as follows:

A. Section a bang area from the recession area on both sides of the head to the back of the frontal plane of the head. Cut the sides using one- (1) finger elevation to the top of the indentation zone. Bring the volume zone down to a stationary guide at the rim zone. The bang is blended at a negative elevation from the top of the nose to the lengths at the side of the head.

B. Section the top panel of the head by laying a comb on top of the head and parting on either side at the point where the comb leaves the head. Beginning at the back of this section, take a 3" (7.6 cm) guide and cut straight across. Use a moving guide while working forward to the bang area. Bring hair in the frontal plane back to this last guide and cut. Blend horizontally on both sides of the top plane.

C. Cut the indentation zone using one- (1) finger elevation throughout. Cut the center panel first using a horizontal guide. Use diagonal partings at the sides, blending the lengths in the front and center back.

D. Cut the center panel in the back of the head from the control zone, and move down to the rim zone using a 3" (7.6 cm) guide from the front of the head. Upon reaching the rim zone, gradually decrease the positive elevation to blend with the nape area. Cut the side sections in the same manner, blending the lengths in the front and center back.

E. Check your cut! Using positive elevation with vertical lines, check and blend from the nape to the crown and then to the front. Using comb control, cut a slight taper along the entire side and back hairline.

F. Using negative elevation, check and blend baseline. Use a Rolling Razor technique to texturize throughout the ends of the hair and create a softer texture.

G. Cut the beard into a round baseline from ear to ear. Begin cutting at the chin and move to the ears. Continue cutting using positive elevation in a rounded form.

H. Finished design with beard.

8. Apply the liquid styling tool of choice to the hair.
9. Airform the hair to create the desired style.
10. Apply finishing spray to hold the completed style.
11. Follow standard clean-up procedures.
12. Document the Client Record/File.

RETAIL RE-BOOK REFERRAL

EVALUATION

GRADE

STUDENT'S NAME

ID#

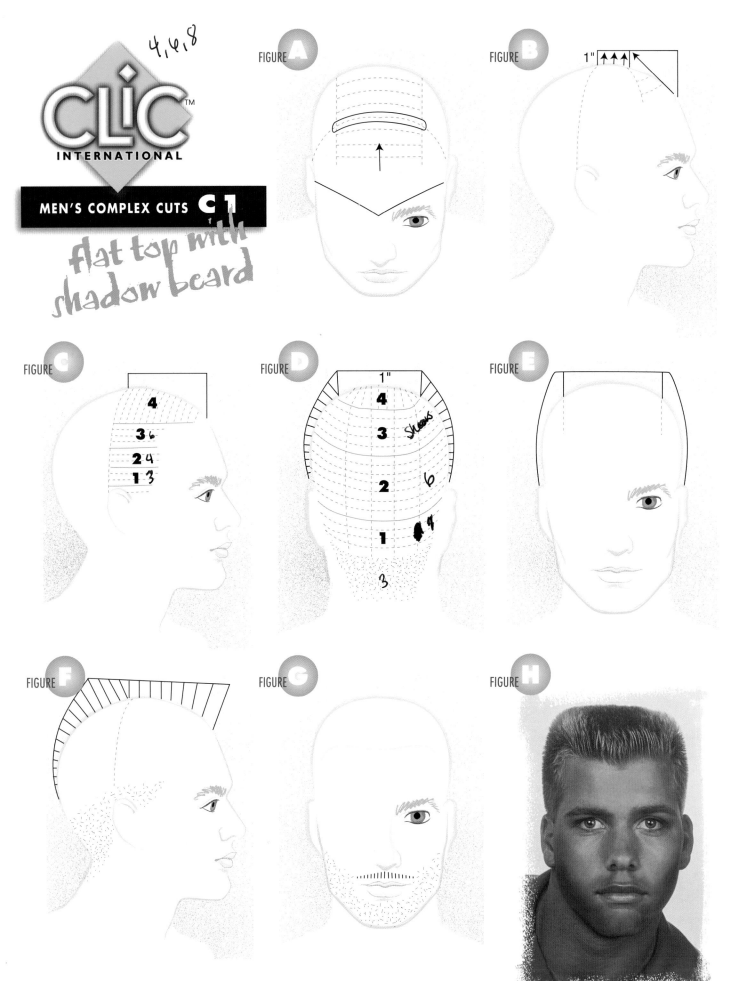

4,6,8

CLiC™
INTERNATIONAL

MEN'S COMPLEX CUTS C1

flat top with shadow beard

FIGURE A

FIGURE B

1"

FIGURE C

4
3 6
2 4
1 3

FIGURE D

1"
4
3 shears
2 6
1 4
3

FIGURE E

FIGURE F

FIGURE G

FIGURE H

Start w/ shortest guard first → same guard for beard

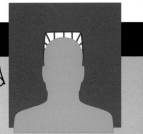
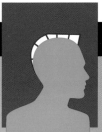

OBJECTIVE

Practice the FLAT TOP, a low-maintenance, squared haircut. This carefree style is cut close from the indentation zone to the crown of the head. It produces a square form. This design is cut using clipper and comb control. The shadow beard is a close clipper cut beard.

TOOLS & MATERIALS

- Neck Strip
- Towels (2)
- Cape
- All-Purpose Brush
- Shampoo
- Shampoo Comb

- Conditioner
- Cutting Comb
- Taper Comb
- Clips
- Standard 5" (12.7 cm) Scissors

- Standard 6" (15.2 cm) Scissors
- Clipper
- Clipper Comb
- Razor
- Trimmer

- Liquid Styling Product
- Airformer
- Brushes
- Finishing Spray
- Client Record Card/File

PROCEDURE

"The Client Consultation is an important part of your professional service. Be sure to complete this step prior to each client service you provide. Your successful retail sales and customer satisfaction rates depend upon it!"

1. Drape the client in preparation for the service.
2. Thoroughly brush the client's hair to remove knots, tangles and hairspray.
3. Cleanse the hair with shampoo. Rinse thoroughly and shampoo again. Rinse.
4. Apply the appropriate conditioning product for the client's needs. Rinse thoroughly and towel dry.
5. Comb the hair to remove tangles.
6. Section the hair for the FLAT TOP and secure it with clips.
7. Perform the haircut as follows:
   A. Section a rectangle on the top of the head from the outside corner of each eye to the back of the head. Cut a guideline 1" (2.5 cm) from the control zone. Hold hair straight up with the comb. The head must be straight and the comb squared with the top of the head. Cut the hair parallel to the floor, moving forward on the head to the back of the frontal area. Then cut the hair parallel to the floor, moving to the back of the head.
   B. Direct hair in the frontal area back to the established length at the frontal area and cut. This creates a length increase to maintain the square top with a frontal extension. Cross check to create a straight line.
   C. Cut the sides using comb control from the ear to the top of the volume zone. Lengths increase moving up the head using the different guards, from 1/4" (0.6 cm) in Area One (1) to 1/2" (1.25 cm) in Area Two (2) and 3/4" (1.9 cm) in Area Three (3). Cut Area Four (4) vertically by holding the comb parallel to the floor and blending the square. Repeat on the other side.
   D. Cut the back in the same manner as the sides. Cut each area from the center to the sides and blend with the front before moving to the next area. Trim the hairline close to the head in the baseline outer perimeter.
   E. Check and blend the sides and top of the head into the square form.
   F. Check and blend the back and top of the head into the square form.
   G. Cut the shadow beard using No. 1 attachment on the clipper. Trim the mustache to blend with the close beard.
   H. Finished design with beard.
8. Apply the liquid styling tool of choice to the hair.
9. Airform the hair to create the desired style.
10. Apply finishing spray to hold the completed style.
11. Follow standard clean-up procedures.
12. Document the Client Record/File.

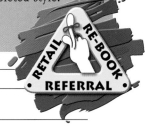

EVALUATION

GRADE

STUDENT'S NAME

ID#

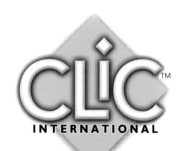

MEN'S COMPLEX CUTS C2

crew cut with mustache

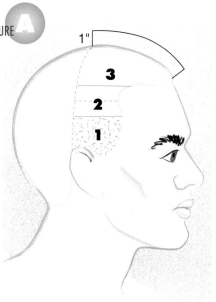

FIGURE A

1"
3
2
1

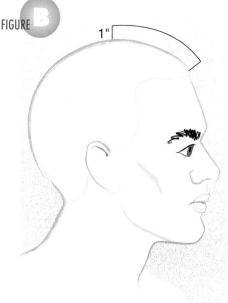

FIGURE B

1"

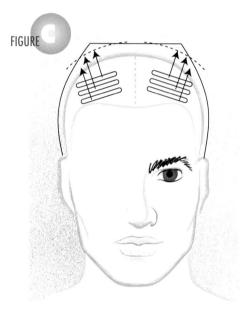

FIGURE C

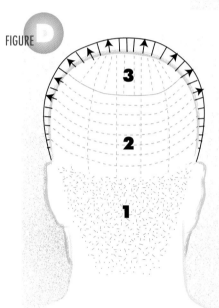

FIGURE D

3
2
1

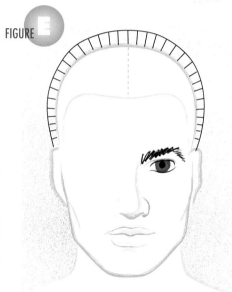

FIGURE E

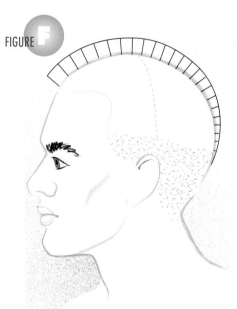

FIGURE F

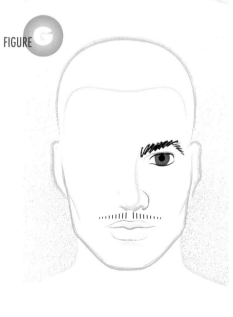

FIGURE G

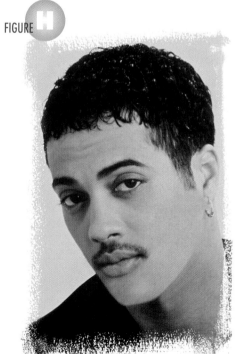

FIGURE H

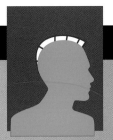

C2 crew cut with mustache

OBJECTIVE

Master the CREW CUT, a no-maintenance style. This short, rounded cut is created using a clipper. The hair is cut close in the nape, and increases to 1" (2.5 cm) on top of the head while conforming to the head shape. The mustache tapers to a point at each side.

TOOLS & MATERIALS

- Neck Strip
- Towels (2)
- Cape
- All-Purpose Brush
- Shampoo
- Shampoo Comb
- Conditioner
- Cutting Comb
- Clips
- Standard 5" (12.7 cm) Scissors
- Standard 6" (15.2 cm) Scissors
- Clipper
- Trimmer
- Razor
- Liquid Styling Product
- Airformer
- Brushes
- Finishing Spray
- Client Record Card/File

PROCEDURE

"The Client Consultation is an important part of your professional service. Be sure to complete this step prior to each client service you provide. Your successful retail sales and customer satisfaction rates depend upon it!"

1. Drape the client in preparation for the service.
2. Thoroughly brush the client's hair to remove knots, tangles and hairspray.
3. Cleanse the hair with shampoo. Rinse thoroughly and shampoo again. Rinse.
4. Apply the appropriate conditioning product for the client's needs. Rinse thoroughly and towel dry.
5. Comb the hair to remove tangles.
6. Section the hair for the CREW CUT and secure it with clips.
7. Perform the haircut as follows:

   A. Cut the side of the head using comb control. Cut Area One (1) 1/8" (0.3 cm) to 1/4" (0.6 cm) to the top of the eyebrow, then increase to 1/4" (0.6 cm) to 1/2" (1.25 cm) in Area Two (2) to the top of the indentation zone. Area Three (3) is cut and blended later.

   B. At the front 1/3 (0.84cm) volume zone, cut a 1" (2.5 cm) center guide in the top panel of the head.

   C. Hold vertical lines straight out from the head and blend the lengths on the sides and the top of the head. Repeat on the other side.

   D. Cut the back of the head in the same manner as the sides. Cut Area One (1) 1/8" (0.3 cm) to

   1/4" (0.6 cm) above the ears. Cut Area Two (2) 1/4" (0.6 cm) to 1/2" (1.25 cm) to the top of the rim zone. Cut the third area using vertical lines, rounding and blending the lengths in the back and the top of the head. Cut all areas from the center to the sides to blend with the front before proceeding to the next area.

   E. Use vertical lines to check and blend the sides.

   F. Same procedure. Use vertical lines to check and make adjustments.

   G. Cut the mustache by first shaving the entire beard except the mustache area. Shave an area between both points on the upper lip, as shown. Shave the mustache clean to create a tapered point on each side. Trim any stray hair.

   H. Finished design with mustache.

8. Apply the liquid styling tool of choice to the hair.
9. Airform the hair to create the desired style.
10. Apply finishing spray to hold the completed style.
11. Follow standard clean-up procedures.
12. Document the Client Record/File.

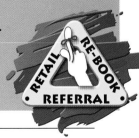

EVALUATION

GRADE

STUDENT'S NAME

ID#

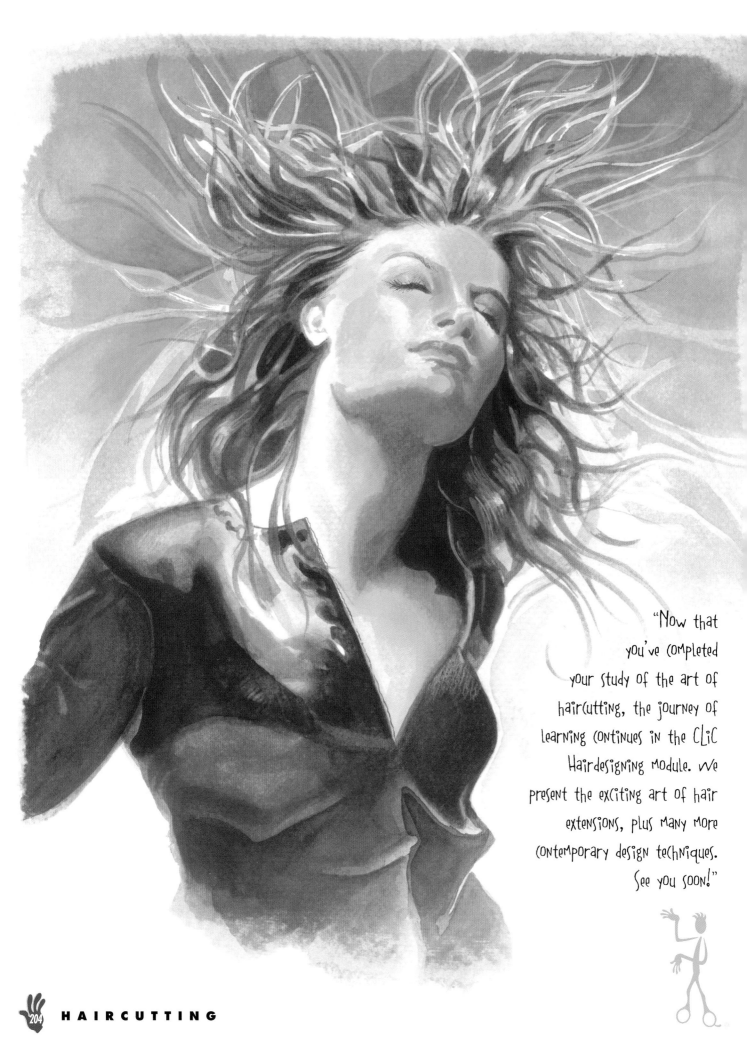

"Now that you've completed your study of the art of haircutting, the journey of learning continues in the CLiC Hairdesigning module. We present the exciting art of hair extensions, plus many more contemporary design techniques. See you soon!"

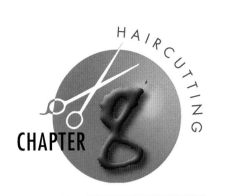

CHAPTER

HAIRCUTTING

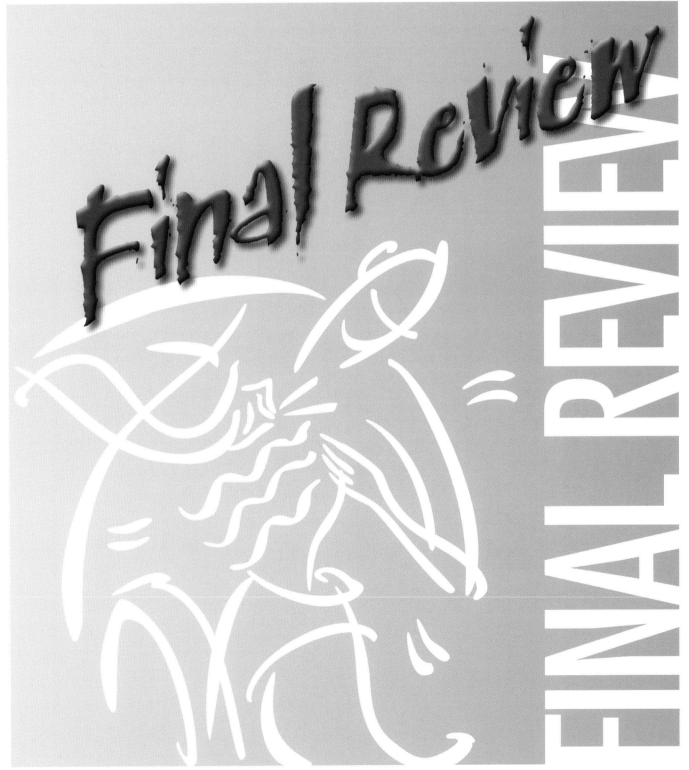

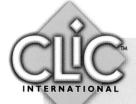

Baseline
Clipper
Convex
Cuticle
Cutting
Damp or wet
Disrupted
Draft
Horizontal
Less
Males
Oval
Plane
Points
Positive
Rim Zone
Shifting
Telogen
Tension
Traveling
Guide

FILL IN THE BLANKS

1. The more teeth per inch that a tapering scissors has, the _____ hair that will be removed.

2. The hair growth cycle consists of anagen, catagen and _____ stages.

3. Lines are created by the shifting of _____.

4. A _____ is the straight area between two points on the curved surface of the head.

5. A _____ moves from one section to another as a reference for the length of additional sections.

6. The air flow from an airformer should follow the natural direction of the _____.

7. _____ is applied to wet hair to stretch it before cutting.

8. _____ need to inherit only one gene for baldness.

9. A _____ line curves outward in an arched shape.

10. _____ elevation is created at levels from 1 to 180 degrees.

11. _____ is moving the hair from its natural growth direction to a different position when cutting.

12. When razor cutting, the hair should be _____.

13. The _____ is considered the perfectly proportioned face shape.

14. _____ lines provide a feeling of width.

15. Textures can be created naturally, chemically or by _____.

16. Positive projection haircuts automatically create a _____ texture.

17. The _____ is the perimeter, outer boundary, design line or fringe line of a hair cut.

18. A _____ is a versatile tool that can be used to remove large quantities of hair in one cut.

19. The _____ is the widest portion of the head where it curves.

20. A _____ is a two-dimensional wet sketch of a finished hair design.

STUDENT'S NAME   DATE   GRADE

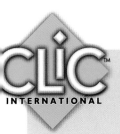

Haircutting FINAL REVIEW QUESTIONS

TRUE OR FALSE

_____ 1. The four corners of the head define the widest part of the fringe and nape areas.

_____ 2. A diagonal line runs in the same direction as the horizon.

_____ 3. You should never lubricate your scissors because it will cause rusting.

_____ 4. The secondary mass is the ball shape on top of the head.

_____ 5. The position of the client's head while cutting does not affect the length of hair.

_____ 6. The scientific method is a standard procedure used to evaluate situations to predict future events.

_____ 7. Dimension is a measurement of length, width and/or depth.

_____ 8. Weave cut scissors are used to remove a very minimal amount of hair.

_____ 9. The triangle is considered the perfect shape because of its structural strength and design balance.

_____10. A stationary guide passes from one section to another.

_____11. Wedge cuts or cuts with stacking are 45 degree cuts.

_____12. Concentric shapes are repeated in different sizes starting from a common starting point.

_____13. While airforming, the elbows should be held into the sides of the body at all times.

_____14. Hair styles with width and volume should be created to counterbalance an oblong face.

_____15. It is not recommended to service male clients with beards because those skills aren't taught in school.

_____16. We can apply the principles of circles and spheres to hair cutting because the head is essentially round.

_____17. Parallel lines travel in different directions.

_____18. The screw of the scissors should face inward when cutting.

_____19. The profiles of the face are described as straight, convex and concave.

_____20. Carpal tunnel syndrome can result from the repeated use of the wrists in an unnatural position.

STUDENT'S NAME
DATE
GRADE

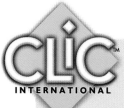

Haircutting FINAL REVIEW QUESTIONS

MULTIPLE CHOICE

1. What type of designs are produced by low elevation haircuts?
   A. light and airy   B. weighted and dense   C. high fashion

2. A design which includes irregular shapes, colors and/or textures which maintain harmony within the overall form is called?
   A. abstract   B. counterbalanced   C. harmonious

3. Which technique provides maximum control and maximum hair removal when razor cutting?
   A. one-finger   B. two-finger   C. three-finger

4. Which shape can be used as a guide to help counterbalance the body proportions?
   A. circle   B. square   C. triangle

5. Which type of line curves inward in a bowl shape?
   A. concave   B. convex   C. curved

6. Negative elevations are cut at which degrees?
   A. 0 degrees   B. 30 degrees   C. 135 degrees

7. Which technique compresses the hair into a common area before it is cut?
   A. squeeze cutting   B. stacking   C. shifting

8. What is used to store photos and/or records of your hair creations?
   A. portfolio   B. folder   C. box

9. The ability to sell by creating the need to buy a service or product is called?
   A. persuasion   B. salesmanship   C. 3-R's

10. What is the term for the study of human body measurements for examination and comparison purposes?
    A. humanology   B. comparatology   C. anthropometry

11. The body, hands and feet must coordinate with what to achieve precision haircuts?
    A. scissors   B. client   C. comb

12. Which direction does the palm face for the palm to scalp cutting technique?
    A. outward   B. inward   C. upward

13. What is created by raising the hair from the head to levels measured in degrees?
    A. volume   B. elevation   C. degrees

14. According to the "3 Parallels of Haircutting," the partings must be parallel to the baseline, the fingers must be parallel to the part and the scissors must be parallel to what?
    A. the fingers   B. the client's head   C. the comb

15. Which technique can be performed on the scalp, center or ends of the hair?
    A. coloring   B. clipper cuts   C. customizing

16. These products help add shine, control and texture to finished hair styles.
    A. liquid tools   B. airformers   C. combs

17. What is the point at the top of the head from which the hair is distributed?
    A. cranial mass   B. control axis   C. base

18. What is the name of a guide that passes from one section to another?
    A. stationary   B. traveling   C. passing

19. What type of partings should be used on thick hair?
    A. thick   B. thin   C. diagonal

20. A haircut that is styled in a disorderly fashion with the appearance of motion and excitement is called:
    A. brush cut   B. bob   C. commotion

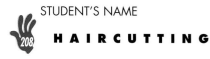

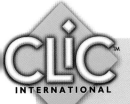

Haircutting FINAL REVIEW QUESTIONS

Asian
Balance
Beards
Blending
Check
Circle
Concentrator
Creativity
Crown
Density
Form
Odd
Outward
Rogaine™
Second Knuckle
Space
Thermal Metal Round
Unbalanced
Progression
Vanishing
Weight Line

FILL IN THE BLANKS

1. _____ scissors are a type of tapering scissors used to create a very fine taper to the hair.

2. A _____ is used to minimize the escape of air from an airformer so that only heat is released.

3. A _____ brush retains heat from the airformer causing the hair to curl faster.

4. _____ lines gradually taper off into infinity.

5. It is very important to _____ the hair as the final stage of each haircut.

6. The harmonious arrangement of the elements of a hair design with nothing emphasized or out of proportion is called _____.

7. The _____ separates low elevated hair from high elevated hair.

8. _____ is a topical hair loss product that is available without a prescription.

9. The palm faces _____ for the palm-to-palm cutting technique.

10. Visually appealing art generally includes _____ design components.

11. The structural outline of a haircut that makes it identifiable is its _____.

12. Never cut beyond the _____ of your middle finger.

13. Hair _____ is typically thinner in the crown, hairline and nape areas.

14. The head is divided into three main components for haircutting: the frontal, _____ and occipital areas.

15. _____ occurs when the design elements of a hairstyle are disproportionate or not well connected.

16. _____ is the ability to develop artistic ideas and concepts using traditional ideas and imagination.

17. _____ between the concentrator on the airformer and the brush will cause bending of the hair and frizz.

18. The density of _____ hair is less than that of Caucasian and African hair.

19. _____ can be used to counterbalance the facial shapes of men.

20. A _____ is actually a series of tangent lines connected at each of the 360 degrees points to create a curved shape.

STUDENT'S NAME   DATE   GRADE

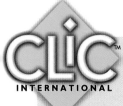
TRUE OR FALSE

_____ **1.** Many texturing techniques create similar effects.

_____ **2.** Stacking is achieved by cutting the hair using high elevation.

_____ **3.** The guard always faces the stylist when razor cutting.

_____ **4.** It is important to cut against the direction of natural growth patterns to minimize difficulty in styling.

_____ **5.** Baselines are created by vertical lines only.

_____ **6.** Never cut more hair than you can control at one time.

_____ **7.** A stationary guide moves from one section to another as a reference for the length of additional sections.

_____ **8.** Scissors should only be cleaned once a month to retain their sharpness and prevent rust.

_____ **9.** To counterbalance is to distribute weight, size, proportion or volume to offset unbalanced proportions and create a harmonious balanced design.

_____ **10.** Vertical lines provide a feeling of width.

_____ **11.** Weave cutting can be performed with a standard scissors using a special technique.

_____ **12.** Art is the skills and techniques used for creative work and learned by observation, study and hands-on experience.

_____ **13.** Single-blade tapering scissors remove more hair than double-blade thinning scissors.

_____ **14.** The volume zone is the lower mass area located below the rim.

_____ **15.** "Getting Planted" is the term for the proper body position for haircutting.

_____ **16.** Customizing textures can only be created with a razor.

_____ **17.** Constructed cuts have heavy ends and minimal action and area also called compact, 0 degree, or one-length cuts.

_____ **18.** The scissors should be perpendicular to the comb when using the scissors-over-comb technique.

_____ **19.** Longer hair styles with volume are recommended for small individuals.

_____ **20.** Sections, sub-sections and partings are used to manage and control defined areas of hair.

Variations of
Women's Cuts

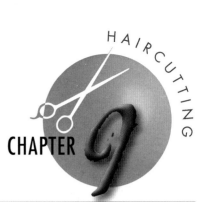

HAIRCUTTING

CHAPTER *9*

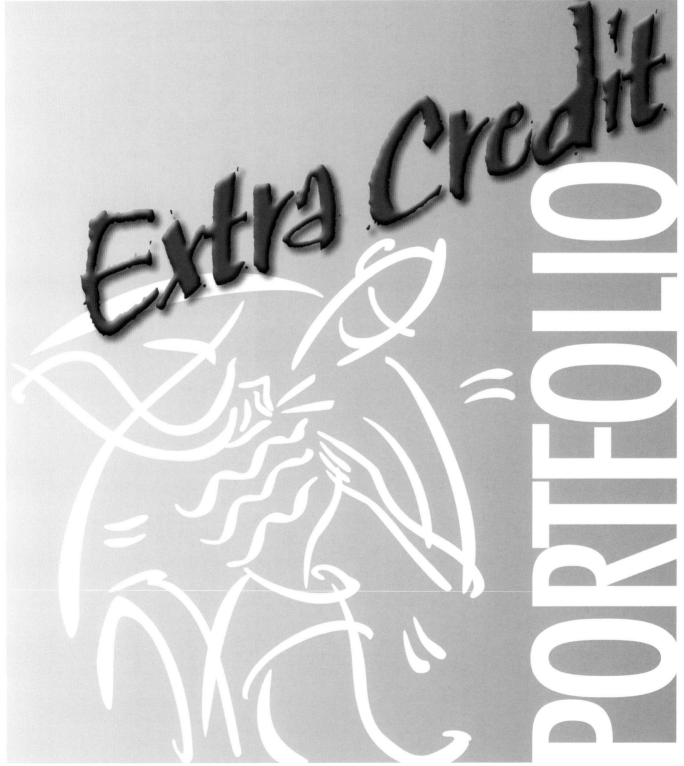

Extra Credit

PORTFOLIO

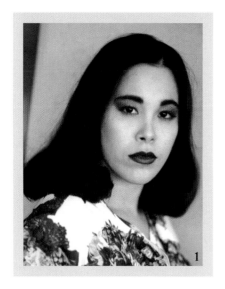

1

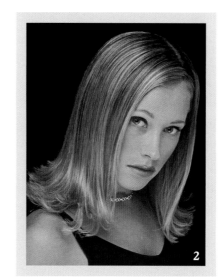

2

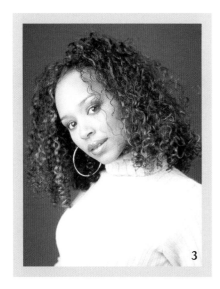

3

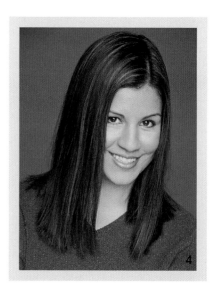

4

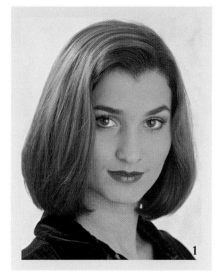

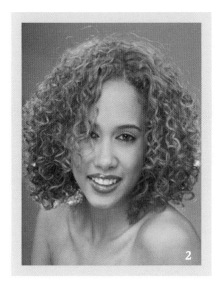

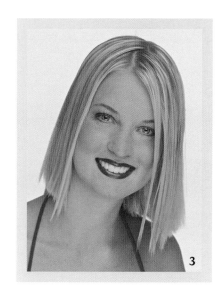

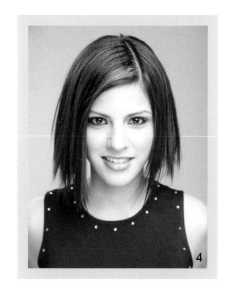

STUDENT'S NAME   DATE   GRADE

Find variations of Career Cut Bob.

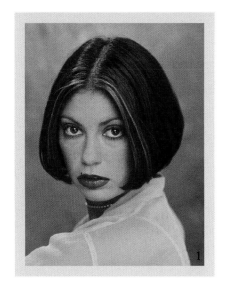

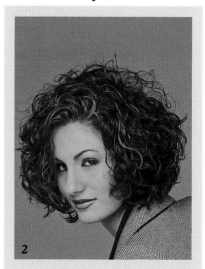

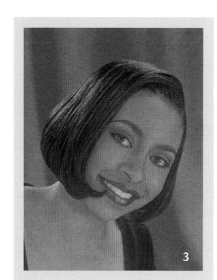

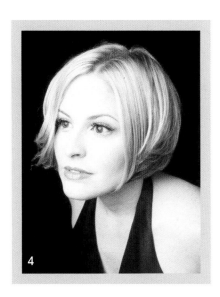

STUDENT'S NAME   DATE   GRADE

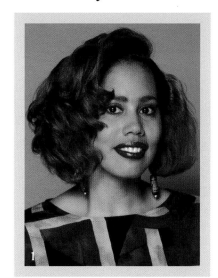

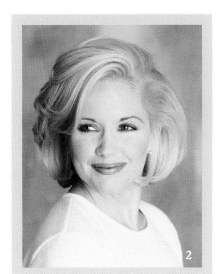

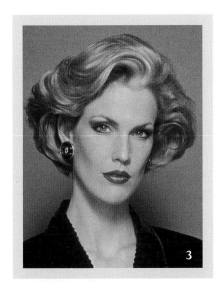

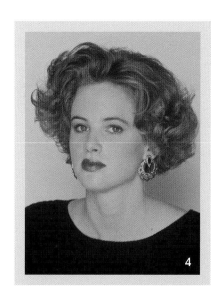

STUDENT'S NAME

DATE

GRADE

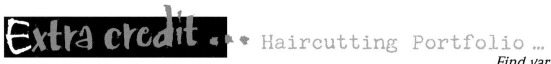

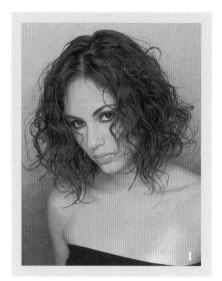

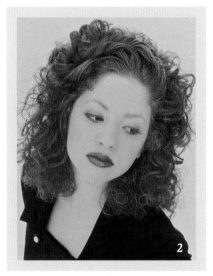

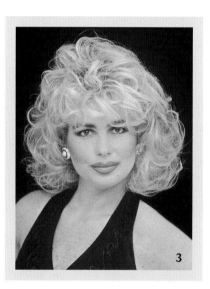

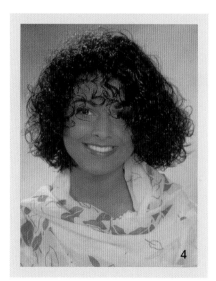

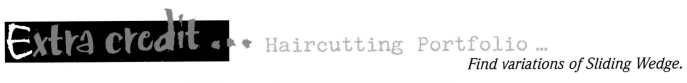

Extra credit

Haircutting Portfolio ...

Find variations of Sliding Wedge.

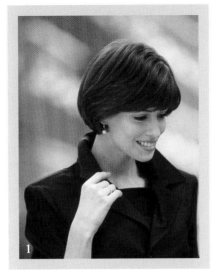

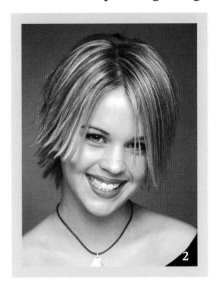

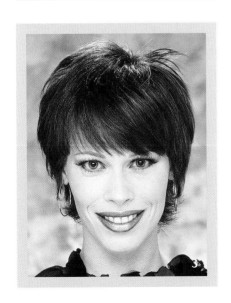

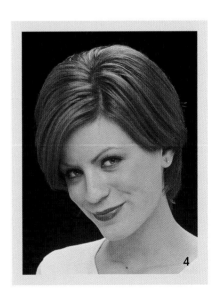

STUDENT'S NAME

DATE

GRADE

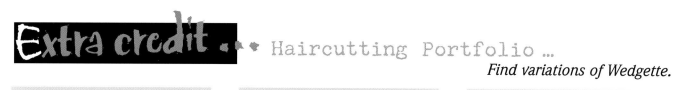

Extra credit ... Haircutting Portfolio ...

Find variations of Wedgette.

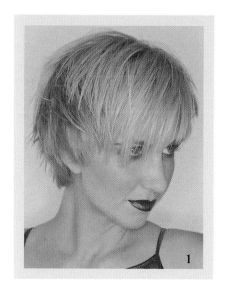

1

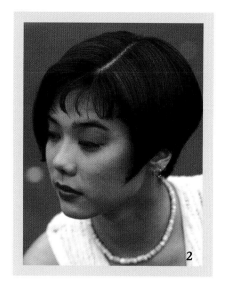

2

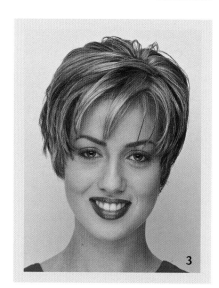

3

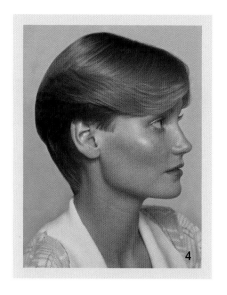

4

STUDENT'S NAME

DATE

GRADE

Find variations of Brush Cut.

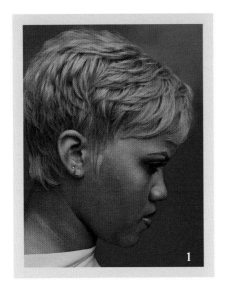

1

2

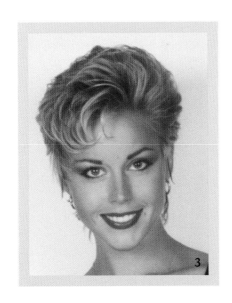

3

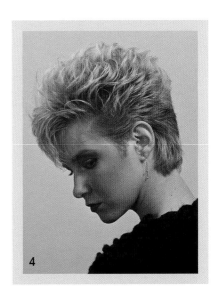

4

Extra credit ... • Haircutting Portfolio ...

Find variations of Fru Fru.

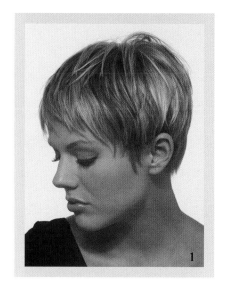

1

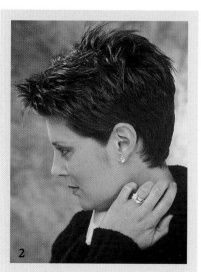

2

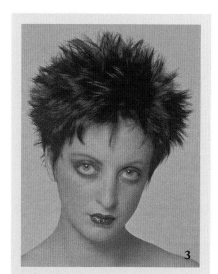

3

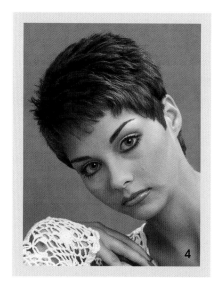

4

STUDENT'S NAME

DATE

GRADE

Find variations of Speed Cut Savage.

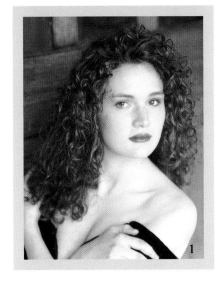

1

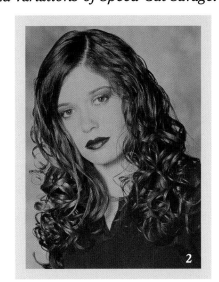

2

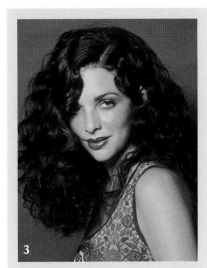

3

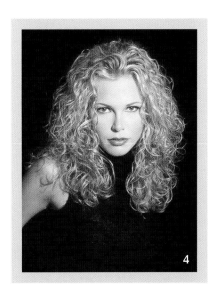

4

STUDENT'S NAME   DATE   GRADE

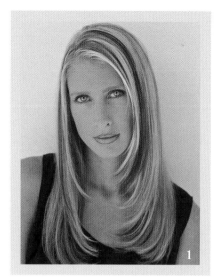
1

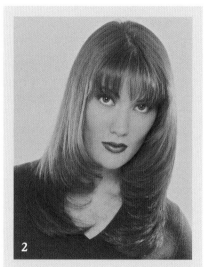
2

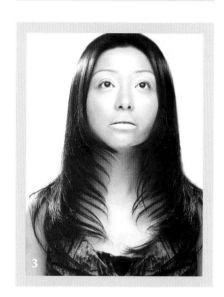
3

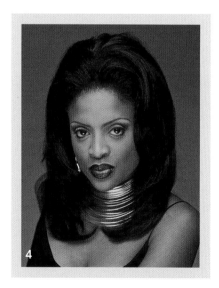
4

Find variations of Boxed Bob.

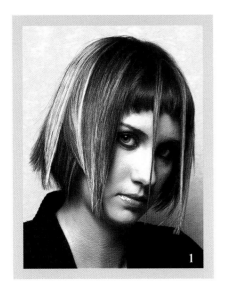

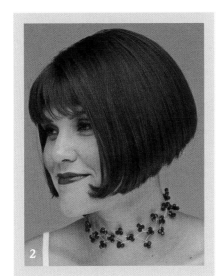

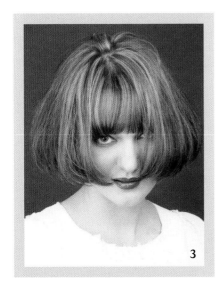

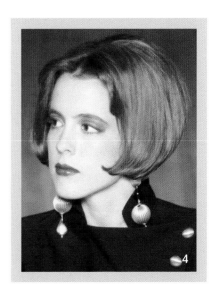

STUDENT'S NAME   DATE   GRADE

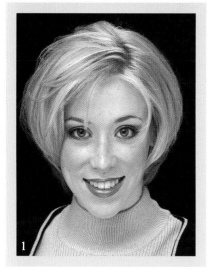

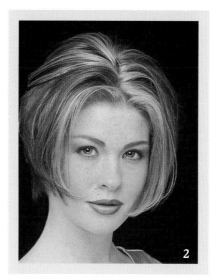

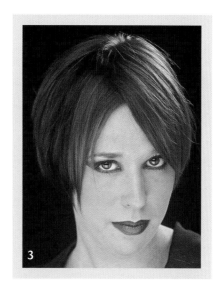

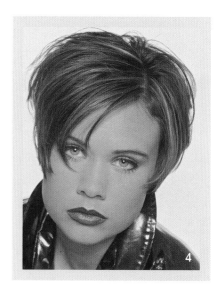

Find variations of Asymmetrical Cut.

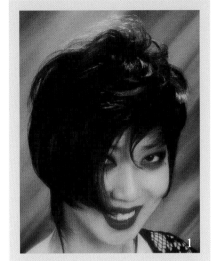
1

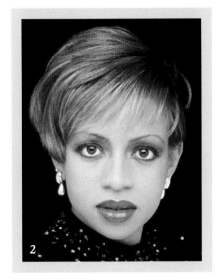
2

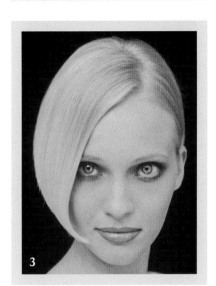
3

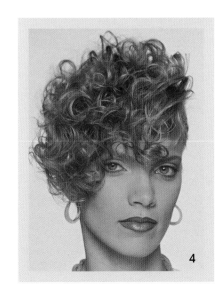
4

STUDENT'S NAME   DATE   GRADE

Extra credit ... • Haircutting Portfolio ...

Find variations of Audacé.

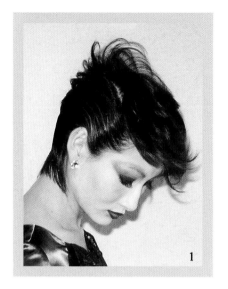

1

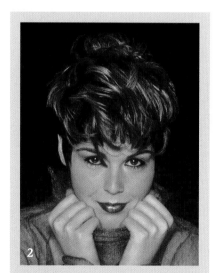

2

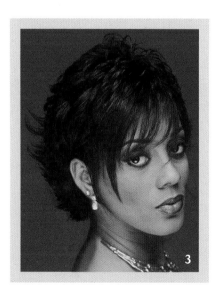

3

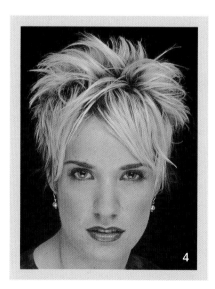

4

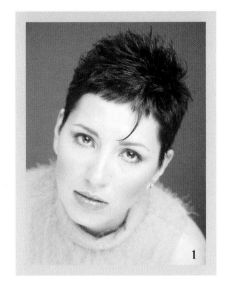

1

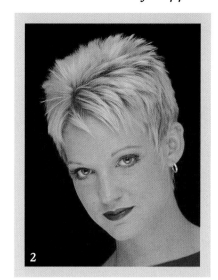

2

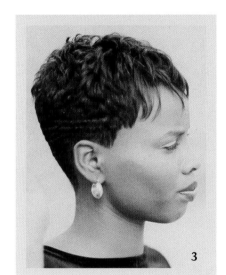

3

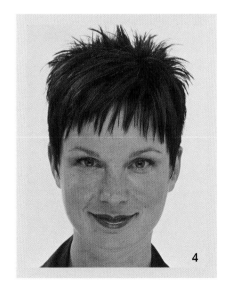

4

STUDENT'S NAME   DATE   GRADE

Haircutting Portfolio ...

Find variations of Creative Clipper.

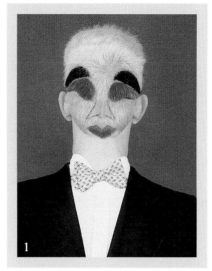

1

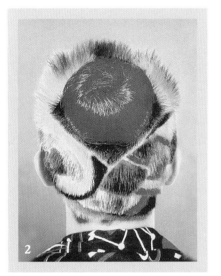

2

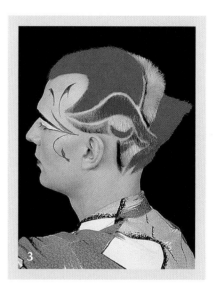

3

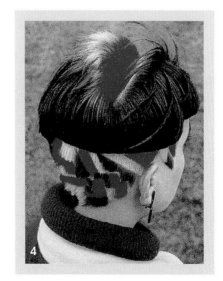

4

STUDENT'S NAME   DATE   GRADE

Female Head Sheet ...

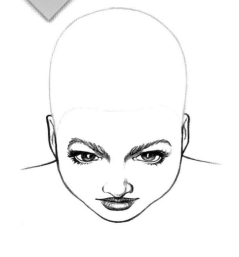

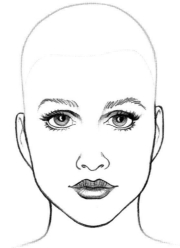

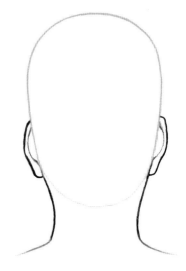

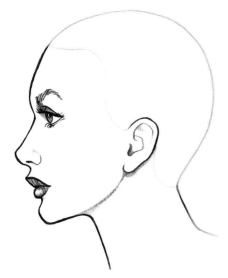

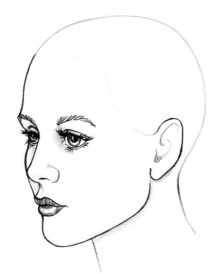

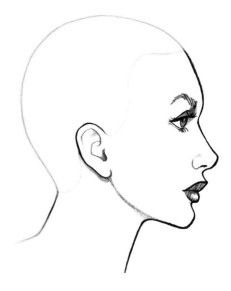

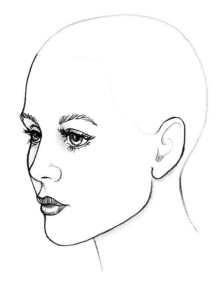

notes... _____

_____

_____

_____

_____

_____

_____

_____

_____

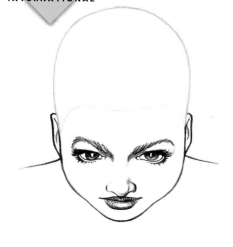
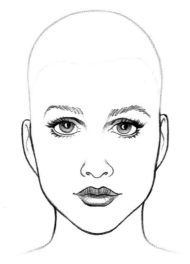
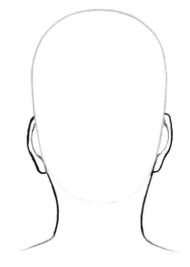

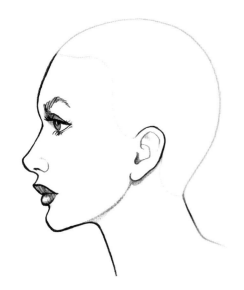
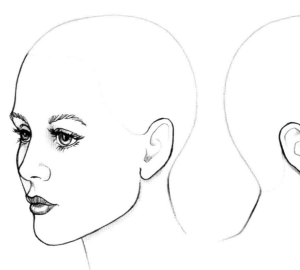

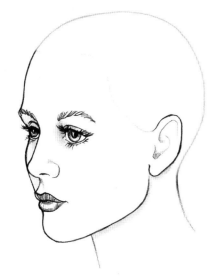

notes...
_____
_____
_____
_____
_____
_____
_____
_____
_____

Variations of
Men's Cuts

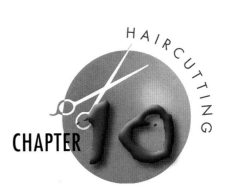

HAIRCUTTING

CHAPTER 10

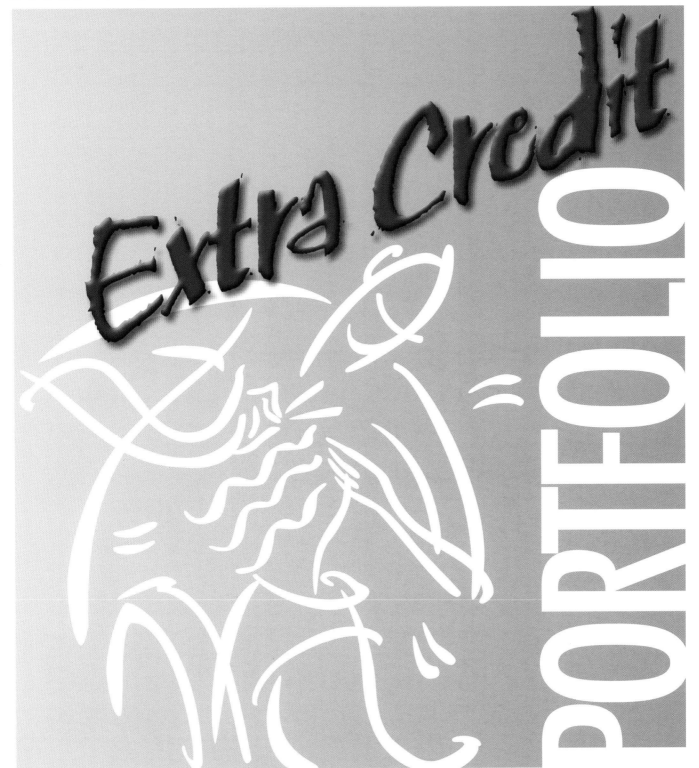

Extra Credit

PORTFOLIO

Find variations of Renegade.

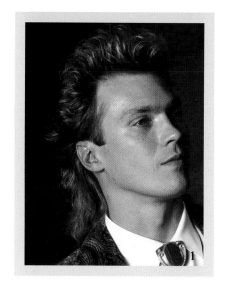

2

3

STUDENT'S NAME   DATE   GRADE

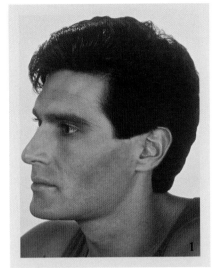

1

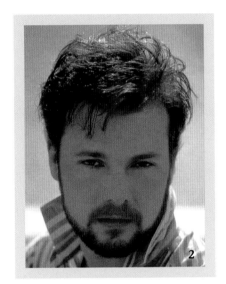

2

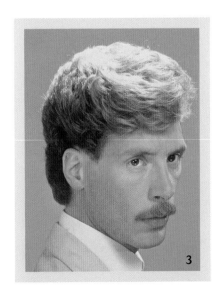

3

STUDENT'S NAME   DATE   GRADE

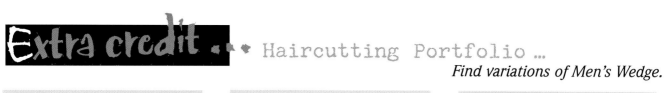

Find variations of Men's Wedge.

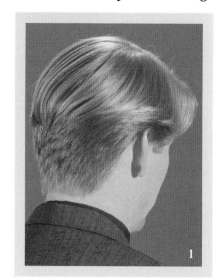

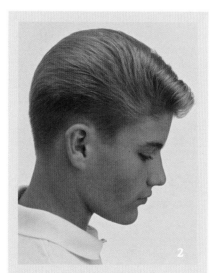

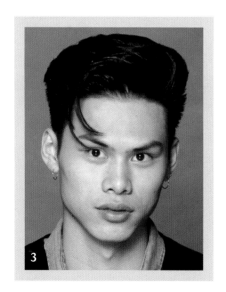

STUDENT'S NAME DATE GRADE

Find variations of Brush Cut.

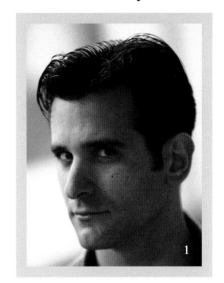

1

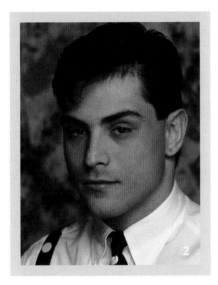

2

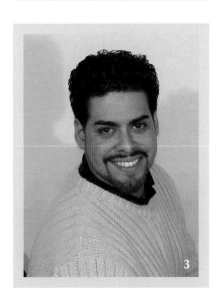

3

STUDENT'S NAME   DATE   GRADE

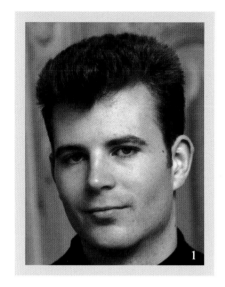

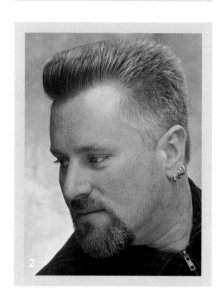

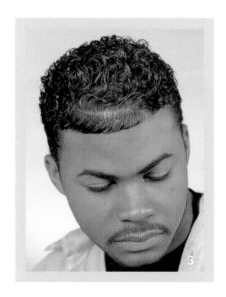

STUDENT'S NAME   DATE   GRADE

Extra credit

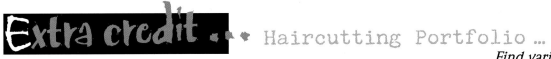

Find variations of Crew Cut.

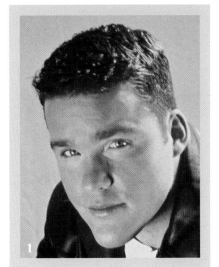

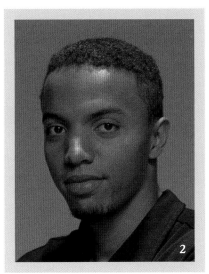

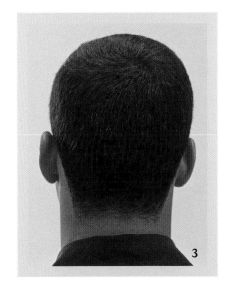

STUDENT'S NAME   DATE   GRADE

CLiC
INTERNATIONAL

Male Head Sheet ...

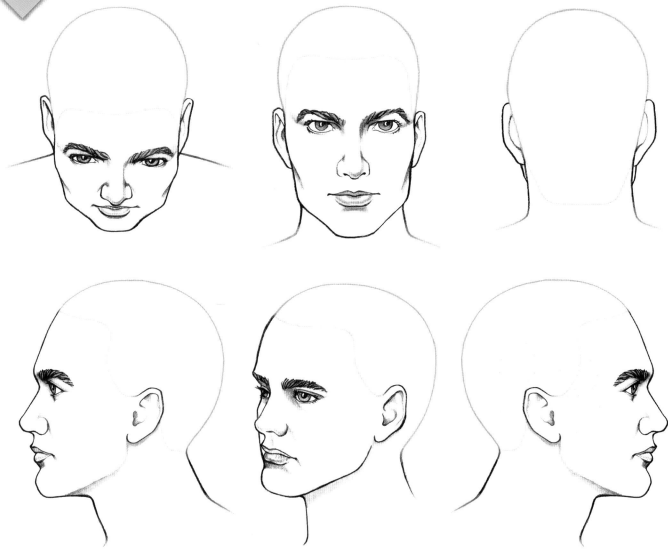

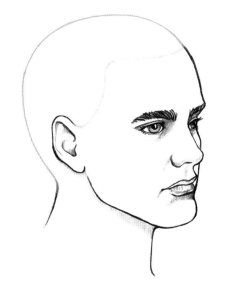

notes... _____

_____

_____

_____

_____

_____

_____

_____

238   **H A I R C U T T I N G**

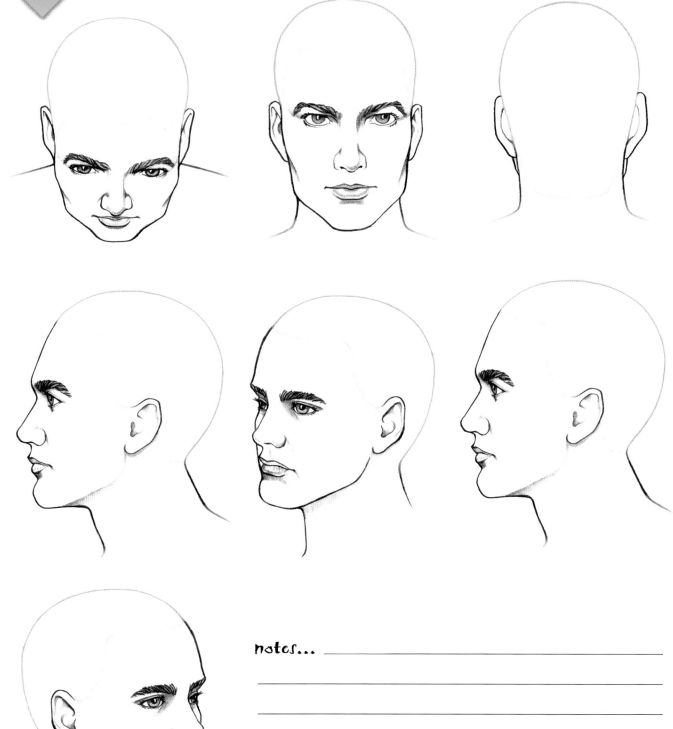

notes... _____

_____

_____

_____

_____

_____

_____

_____

_____

Index...

A

Abstract, 14
Adjustable scissors, 37
African hair, 77
Air diffuser, 53
Airforming, 50–55
Angles, 14, 101
Anthropometry, 14, 70
Architectural haircutting, 98–99
Art, 15
Asian hair, 77
Asymmetrical cut, 182–183
Audacé, 184–185

B

Backcombing, 149
Balance, 15
Baldness, 80–81
Baseline, 104
Beards, 92–93
    renegade, 192–193
    rounded, 198–199
    shadow, 200–201
    square, 196–197
Blending scissors, 36
Blow drying, 50–55
Bob
    boxed, 178–179
    career, 160–161
    disrupted, 180–181
    forward fringe, 176–177
    page, 156–157
    speed cut, 158–159
Body shape, 72–73
    counterbalances for, 86
Boundaries, 16
Boxed bob, 178–179
Brush cut, 170–171, 198–199
Brushes, airforming, 54–55
Butterfly clips, 56

C

Career bob, 160–161
Curved funnel finger comb, 33
Caucasian hair, 77
Center area customizing, 144
Chemical textures, 140
Clamps, 56
CLiC Cutting (C.C.C.) Concept, 132–151

Clippette cut, 186–187
Clipper comb, 33
Clipper cuts, 188–189
Clippers, 46–49, 63, 66
Clips, 56
Combination lines, 101
Combs, 30–33
Computer tools, 60–61
Concave lines, 16, 103
Concentric, 17
Conflict, 17
Connecting lines, 106–107
Constructed, 17
Control axis, 18
Control zone, 18
Conventional airformer, 52
Convex lines, 16, 103
Counterbalance, 15, 86
    with beards, 92–93
    for body shape, 86
    for facial shape, 87–91
Creative clipper cuts, 188–189
Creativity, 18
Crew cut, 202–203
Crowns, 78
Curved lines, 103
Customized textures, 144–151
Cut and tapering scissors, 37
Cuticle scraping, 149
Cutting. See Haircutting
Cutting accessories, 57
Cutting collar, 57
Cutting lines, 104
Cutting lotion, 59
Cutting techniques, 19
Cutting textures, 140–151

D

Degrees of cutting, 20, 110–113
Density, 20
Design, 20
Detanglers, 58
Diagonal direction, 21
Diagonal lines, 24, 102
Diagram, 20
Diffuser airformer, 52
Dimension, 21
Direction, 21
Disconnected, 22
Disposable razor trimmer, 45
Disrupted bob, 180–181
Disruption cutting, 146
Double blade thinning scissors, 37

Draft, 22
Duckbill clips, 56

E

Edges, 22
Elevations, 19, 108–109, 122–123
End area customizing, 144
Even progression, 116

F

Facial shape, 82–85
    counterbalances for, 87–91
Finger comb, 33
Fingertip razor, 44
Finishing spray, 58
Flat top, 200–201
Form, 22
45 degree cuts, 111
Forward fringe bob, 176–177
Free stylin', 23
Fru fru, 172–173
Functional cuts, 23

G

Gels, 58
Glazes, 58
Guide + distance = length theory, 114–115
Guideline, 104
Guides, 23

H

Hair
    density of, 79
    growth patterns of, 78
    shape of, 76
    texture of, 27, 140–151
Haircutting. See also Cutting
    architectural, 98–99
    C.C.C. Concept for, 132–151
    coordination and control of, 94–95
    degrees of, 110–113
    flow chart for, 120–121
    line construction in, 100–107
    mathematics of, 98–127
    problem-solving in, 130–131
    science of, 130–151
    seven steps of, 118–119
Haircutting tools, 29–68
Hairlines, 78
Hair loss, 80–81
Hair pick, 53

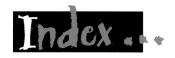

Index ...

Extra Credit ...

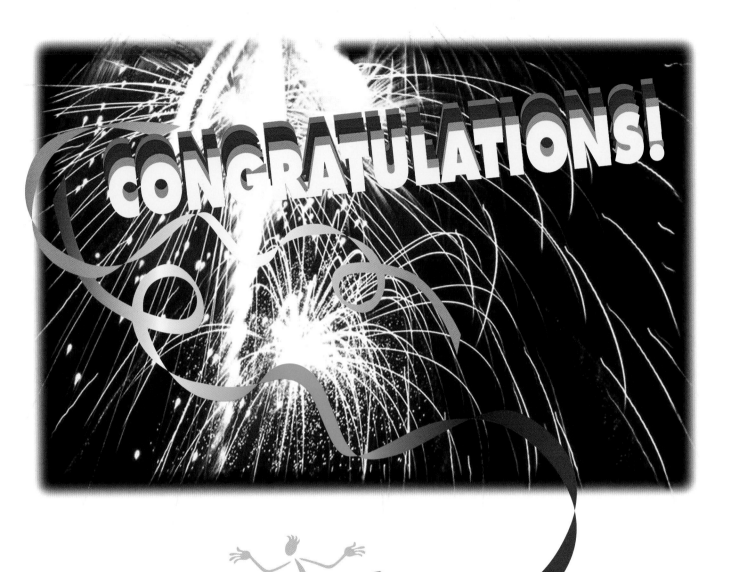

CONGRATULATIONS!

"I knew you could do it!
There sure is a lot to learn about haircutting, isn't there?
The new knowledge you have acquired is just the beginning.
Through continuous investigation and experimentation, you'll
be able to perform precision haircutting services!"

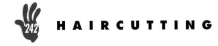

CLiC Classmates Sign In ...

School _____   Class of _____

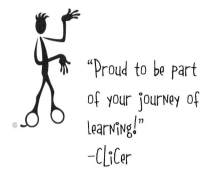

"Proud to be part
of your journey of
learning!"
-CLiCer

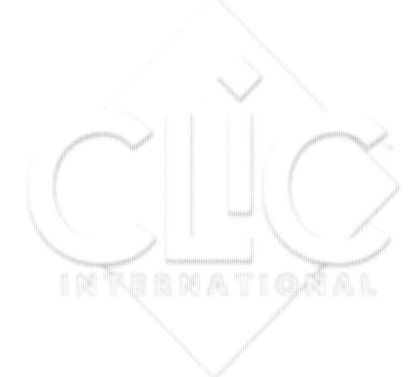

Thank you for joining our professional team of great haircutters!

 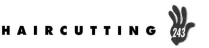

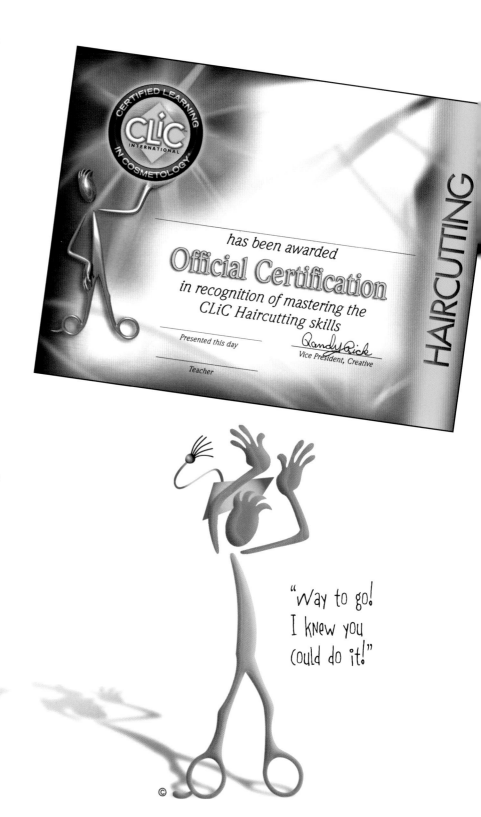

CONGRATULATIONS!

Now that you have completed your journey through the **Haircutting** module, you are ready to take the Student Certification Exam. With a passing grade, you will receive official certification documenting that you have mastered the skills presented in the **Haircutting** module.

As you continue on your journey through each of the **CLiC** learning modules, you will receive a certificate for each module completed successfully. After completing all modules with passing grades, you will receive a **CLiC** masters certification award.

Best of success to you!

For more information call:
CLiC INTERNATIONAL®
1.800.207.5400
www.clicusa.com

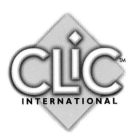

"Way to go! I knew you could do it!"

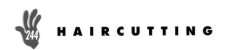

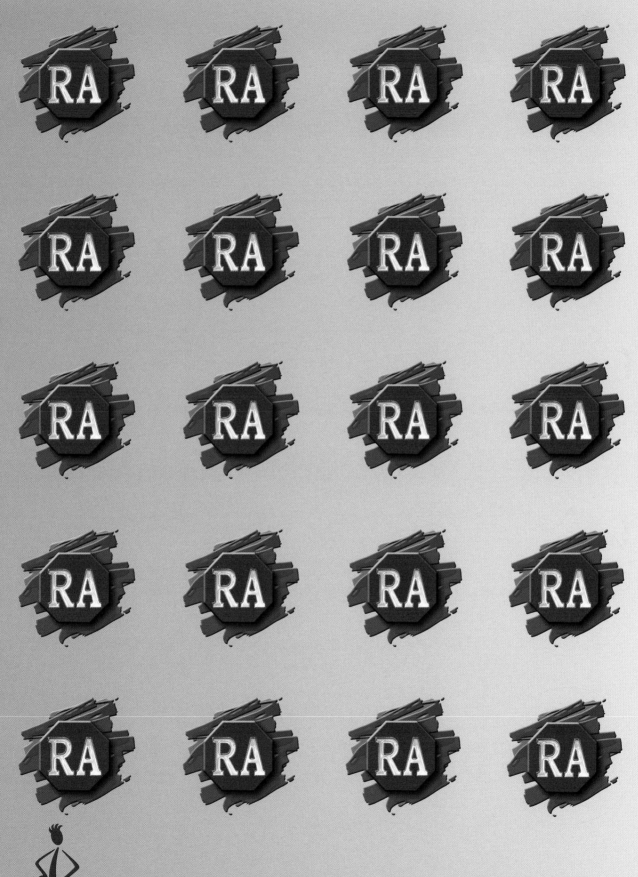

"Here are the stickers we talked about on page 9. Your instructor will help you learn which regulatory issues occur in your area."